1:59

*SPECIAL THANKS TO CORALEE THOMPSON, MD
FOR HER ESSENTIAL EDITING AND TECHNICAL INPUT.*

1:59

THE SUB-TWO-HOUR MARATHON IS WITHIN REACH—HERE'S HOW IT WILL GO DOWN, AND WHAT IT CAN TEACH ALL RUNNERS ABOUT TRAINING AND RACING

DR. PHILIP MAFFETONE

WITH BILL KATOVSKY

Skyhorse Publishing

Skyhorse Publishing books may be purchased in bulk at special discounts for sales promotion, corporate gifts, fund-raising, or educational purposes. Special editions can also be created to specifications. For details, contact the Special Sales Department, Skyhorse Publishing, 307 West 36th Street, 11th Floor, New York, NY 10018 or info@skyhorsepublishing.com.

Skyhorse® and Skyhorse Publishing® are registered trademarks of Skyhorse Publishing, Inc.®, a Delaware corporation.

Visit our website at www.skyhorsepublishing.com.

10 9 8 7 6 5 4 3 2 1

Library of Congress Cataloging-in-Publication Data is available on file.

Cover design by Brian Peterson
Cover photo © Rex Features via AP Images

Print ISBN: 978-1-62914-817-5
Ebook ISBN: 978-1-62914-837-3

Printed in the United States of America

CONTENTS

INTRODUCTION

Why couldn't Pheidippides have died at 20 miles?

—FRANK SHORTER, 1972 Olympic
marathon gold medalist

The two-hour marathon barrier will be broken. It should happen soon. There is widespread consensus in the running community, including coaches, exercise researchers, and elite marathoners, that a 1:59 marathon is entirely possible. Where opinions differ, however, is exactly when it will occur. Many claim that it will happen within a decade or perhaps longer. Others maintain that the record won't take place in our lifetime. I am much more optimistic. I believe that a 1:59 will happen within the next several years, maybe even earlier. That's primarily because the human body is now capable of making this historical leap forward.

The current world record stands at 2:03:23. Wilson Kipsang, of Kenya, set it at the 2013 Berlin Marathon. Kipsang is just the latest in a talented group of East African distance runners who have been steadily chipping away at the marathon record in recent years. Another Kenyan, Geoffrey Mutai, won the 2011 Boston Marathon by the narrowest of margins, out-dueling fellow countryman Moses Mosop to win by a scant four seconds. His time, 2:03:02, easily beat the world record of 2:03:59 set three years earlier at the Berlin Marathon by Ethiopia's Haile Gebrselassie. While Mutai's time was the fastest ever for the marathon, the international governing body for running disqualified the time as an official world record because the race went point-to-point on an overall downhill course.

Each time there's a new world record, the media use the occasion to rekindle speculation about running's final, most challenging, and tantalizing barrier: the sub-two-hour marathon. Who will become that first runner to go 1:59 and become universally celebrated as marathon's Roger Bannister? Will it be a Kenyan, Ethiopian, American, or someone from another country?

Three minutes isn't very long. It's about the time it takes to read this page and the next, or soft-boil an egg. Yet elite marathoners seemed to have reached a plateau in running significantly faster. Ever since 26.2 miles was made the official marathon distance over a century ago, world-record times have been steadily dropping. The American runner John Hayes was the marathon's original world-record holder after clocking 2:55:18 at the 1908 London Olympics. By 1920, over twenty minutes had been shaved off this time. Following the Second World War, elite runners lowered the marathon record to 2:15 by the end of the 1950s. This decrease was attributed to rigorous year-round training.

As the first major running boon took hold in the 1960s, times descended even further to 2:08. Then the pace of new world-record times slowed. While times have continued to drop—in the past 15 years, eight world records have been set on Berlin's flat and fast marathon course—it took 25 years for three-and-a-half minutes to be trimmed off the record. (Ethiopia's Belayneh Dinsamo's clocked 2:06:50 at the 1988 Rotterdam Marathon in the Netherlands.)

If one looked at the fastest marathon times of recent years, it's perfectly fair to ask the following: Will it take another quarter of a century to see the world-record mark dip below two hours?

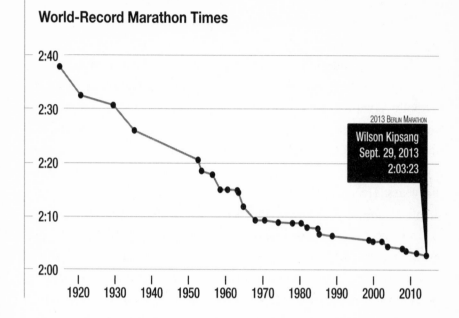

World-Record Marathon Times

2013 BERLIN MARATHON
Wilson Kipsang
Sept. 29, 2013
2:03:23

Several distinguished running stars of the past agree that yes, a runner will one day go sub-two hours. England's two-time Olympic gold middle-distance great Sebastian Coe recently told BBC Radio, "Go down to your local running track, run a lap in under 70 seconds, and then continue for 105 laps. You get the scale of what we are talking about. The arithmetic of a sub-two-hour marathon is both instructive and quite sobering. You've got to run four minutes, 35 seconds per mile over the course."

Bannister, now eighty-four, who was the first person to run a sub-four-minute mile—it happened sixty years ago on a gravel track in Oxford, England—offered this additional perspective: "[The runner] needs a course that is relatively flat, without hills. He needs a freedom from wind because that slows you down and he has to have pacemakers who will enable him to relax."

Alberto Salazar, who won the 1981 New York City Marathon in 2:08:13, then a world record, now spends most of his time in Oregon coaching top elite runners for Nike, including Mo Farah, who is the current 10,000 meters Olympic and World champion and 5,000 meters Olympic, World, and European champion. Despite meticulously preparing Farah for the next chapter in the Somali-born British citizen's storied running career—the marathon (Farah finished eighth at the London 2014 race in 2:08:21)—Salazar does not think that a sub-two hour marathon will happen in the coming years. He told the national radio show *Here and Now* that he's skeptical about just how much faster the 26.2-mile race can be run. "I don't believe [it's possible] in our lifetime, [with] the human body as it is right now. I don't see the marathon going under two hours."

Dr. Michael Joyner, an anesthesiologist and exercise researcher at the Mayo Clinic in Rochester, Minnesota, who has long been a student of human endurance, is more bullish about the sub-two hour breakthrough. Joyner was the author of the first published scientific paper to address how fast a human body could possibly run 26.2 miles. The study, which appeared in 1991 in the *Journal of Applied Physiology*, came to the conclusion that it was theoretically possible to clock 1:57:58.

What then will it take for an elite distance runner to reach 1:59? This accomplishment will require more than raw talent, optimal body size, and the right kind of athletic genes. There are many other important factors to consider: better diet, avoidance of overtraining, living high and training low, improved fat-burning or aerobic efficiency, increased running economy, proper rest and recovery, harnessing the untapped potential of the racing brain, the right kind of shoes (or even going barefoot!), and having marathoners race on a one-mile loop.

Each of the above topics is covered in detail in this book. For running enthusiasts everywhere, the information will give you an art- and science-based understanding of the true potential of human endurance. And in turn, you can apply the same principles outlined in these pages to your own running, whether it's seeking a **PR** in the 10K, half-marathon, marathon, or ultra-marathon.

This book is also somewhat of a departure from my previous books. Writing it has allowed me to take a look back at the running boom, the downward trend of marathon times, and all the factors that could help a runner go 1:59. While I have continued to write and lecture about endurance sports, kept abreast with the latest research, and occasionally consult, I no longer run a large clinic, where many athletes came for training and treatment. For the past fifteen years, I've been away from the day-to-day work with runners, and this has given me a different perspective of the sport. Getting out of the trenches, so to speak, has allowed me to arrive at a more objective view of the likelihood of a 1:59 marathon. This critical detachment, and liberation from any particular bias, has made me even more confident that a sub-two hour marathon will happen soon. That is why I wrote this book.

—Dr. Philip Maffetone
Oracle, Arizona

CHAPTER 1

TIME

The marathon is the focal point of all that has gone before and all that will come afterward.

—DR. GEORGE SHEEHAN

Runners are obsessed with time. They fixate on their own personal bests, past finishing times dating back years, training and racing splits, and of course, world records. One of the main reasons there is little agreement, if not serious doubt about the likelihood of a sub-two hour marathon happening any time soon, is that the current debate often mistakenly focuses on the notion of time in isolation of other factors that might influence the final outcome.

The 1:59 marathon may turn out to be 1:59:50, 1:59:59, or some combination of numbers that will seem almost irrelevant, not unlike Bannister's sub-four-minute mile. Ask most runners about that most famous of sporting records and they will know it was three minutes and fifty-something seconds (it was officially 3:59.4). Even the title of Bannister's own memoir is *The Four-Minute Mile*.

There's another reason why I refer to "1:59" rather than "2:00." That's because if the discussion dwells on "2" and not "1," the brain is actually affected by a misapplication of mental visualization. As I will show in the chapter on the brain, this organ is the marathoner's most powerful instrument. The brain needs to know that it can go

1:59. It needs to formulate an indelible picture of 1-5-9, and not 2-0-0. The highly trained and healthy body will follow the brain's instruction.

MAKING HEADLINES

The photo of Roger Bannister's record-setting mile finish shows several track officials peering down at their hand-held stopwatches. Now everything is computerized, and so when a runner does run that sub two-hour marathon, one can assume that the photo that will be viewed everywhere in newspapers, magazines, social-media feeds, and blogs will be that of the marathoner joyfully standing next to a large electronic display showing 1:59 and various seconds.

Unfortunately, many of those in the running world, from coaches to scientists to journalists and even athletes themselves, are gripped by what I call "two-hour-marathonitis." This affliction is characterized by an over-reliance of number crunching and super-detailed comparisons of past times in an attempt to question whether going under two hours for the marathon is even possible. It's enough to make one's head spin in confusion.

Let's consider one example of this obsession with stats and numbers. Here's an excerpt from an article by *Runner's World*'s Scott Douglas, "Why a Sub-2:00 Marathon Won't Happen Soon," which appeared online within days of Wilson Kipsang's 2013 world-record time of 2:03:23.

Kipsang lowered the record by 15 seconds, or approximately .57 seconds per mile. If someone were to lower the mile world record from its current 3:43.14 by .57 seconds to 3:42.57, no one would think, "Gosh, a 3:34.79 mile is just around the corner!"

But that's the equivalent of what's happening with the sub-2:00 marathon talk. The record being lowered by .57 seconds per mile is taken to suggest that reducing it down by another 7.78 seconds per mile (204 seconds divided by 26.2 miles) will happen soon.

To further put into perspective what taking 7.78 seconds per mile off a record means, consider that doing so would lower the 5000-meter world record from 12:37 to 12:13, the 10,000-meter mark from 26:17 to 25:29, and the half marathon record from 58:23 to 56:41. Those times might come someday, but nobody knowledgeable about distance running talks as if they're near-future certainties.

I am sure Mr. Douglas means well, but he, like many others, totally misses looking at the larger picture. Differentiating between marathon times and those times achieved in shorter events is critical; otherwise, one undervalues the overall relationship between pace and energy. So making comparisons between shorter distances and 26.2 miles is not even physiologically appropriate. It's also the reason that younger elites tend to excel in shorter events, while maturity later allows them to become more accomplished marathoners. Pacing is an acquired skilled, honed by years of racing experience.

There is a powerful component of aerobic fitness involved in the marathon. For 26.2 miles, the body obtains 99 percent of its energy from the aerobic system. The mix of important fuels—from both glucose and body fat—is different than that used during running shorter races, when more anaerobic power is required. In the mile, aerobic and anaerobic contributions are 60 and 40 percent, respectively. Aerobic energy contributions, with reduced anaerobic need, rise quickly to about 88 percent for the 5K and 90 percent for 10K.

Training to run a faster marathon is made possible because you can influence the aerobic system much more than you can anaerobic power, where genetics have a greater role. In other words, the shorter, anaerobic-based, speedier events employ more genetic features of the runner—much less so in a marathon. It's like the old saying, *sprinters are born and endurance athletes are made.*

In later chapters, I discuss how the body can better harness its own plentiful supply of aerobic endurance, in combination, to a lesser degree, with its limited reserves of anaerobic power. This is all related to one's running economy, and is important to know whether you're a first-time marathoner or a sub-2:10 runner.

TRAINING TIME

One of the reasons why some physiologists, coaches, and athletes don't rely on the traditional VO_2max test—the maximal oxygen uptake—is time. During a VO_2max treadmill evaluation, the runner is neither told how long to run nor miles necessary, only that he or she will continue running to exhaustion, or some maximum level. Without this critical information, the brain does not know how to optimally proceed in making the body run; consequently, the test results are less valid.

Our running culture traditionally trains by miles or kilometers. Hardly anyone goes out for a workout without knowing beforehand, and with a fair degree of accuracy, how long a distance the run will be. Specific mileage programs appear in magazines, are prescribed by coaches, and prepared by athletes as if running a certain number of miles means something very precise. It does not.

Our current race culture essentially does the same thing. Almost all events are promoted by a specific distance—5K, 10K, half-marathon, a marathon. Nervously standing or crouching, and maybe shuffling in place at the front of the starting line, elite runners intently focus on time. Many have their index fingers gently resting on their watches' start button, waiting for the gun to go off. Mid-packers do the same, as much focused on a precisely calculated and anticipated finishing time as anything else during the course of the race. (Stand near the finish line of a marathon, and you'd be surprised by just how many runners look first at their watches as they cross the finish.)

But independent of the timepiece and occurring deep inside the brain, all the miles are being mentally processed. It's natural for us to do that. The brain needs to know how much time it has to accomplish the task at hand. That's because time is transcendent. It defines who and what we are.

As a coach, I always used time, and not miles, when writing up programs for my athletes. I found that many runners initially had difficulty adapting to my approach. Even when they were weaned off the notion of miles, they still wanted to refer to, say, a one-hour run as going a certain number of miles. Often they kept these secrets to themselves, but in their diaries, which I often looked at, they were jotted down in minutes and hours.

Finally, in order to make each timed workout much more meaningful, one's heart rate should also be included in a training log. Simply writing down "ran seven miles" merely indicates how far the run was, and little more.

Smarter, more efficient training may be just one of the reasons that we are now witnessing breakthrough marathon times. These appear as personal bests by individual runners, with numbers that get lost in the dense fog of statistics. In 2011, Kenyan Patrick Makau ran a record time of 2:03:38 in Berlin. While many focus on the record being broken by "only" twenty-one seconds, it was a PR for Makau by a minute and ten seconds. American Ryan Hall, who had a relatively poor showing in the 2014 Boston Marathon, had run a personal best three years earlier on the same course by a minute and nineteen seconds (2:04:58). Just ahead of him was Ethiopian Gebre Gebremariam, who ran his all-time best by just over three minutes. We rarely see such significant breakthroughs in times during shorter events on this elite level, even those that are percentage-based, wind-aided, or on fast road courses.

Despite the statistician's meta-analysis, whereby the trickle-down effect is used to show that marathon records are broken by some predictable pattern and usually not by very large differences, this is not always the case. Certainly there are several instances of marathon records being set in which a runner knocks down a huge chunk of time—thirty or forty-five seconds—from the previous world best. In 1967, Australian Derek Clayton's 2:09:36 was almost two-and-a-half minutes faster than the previous world best run by Japan's Morio Shigematsu at 2:12:00 (1965). Looking back further, the UK's Jim Peters ran 2:18:40 in 1953 to break his one-year-old marathon record of 2:20:42. The previous record was 2:25:39, run by Korea's Suh Yun-bok in 1947—making Peters' world-best margin seven minutes and change, or about five percent.

A more accurate gauge of the progression of world-record times is by looking at *percentage improvements*. To run 1:59, a runner would have to break the current world record by 3.2 percent, and even less using Geoffrey Mutai's unofficial Boston marathon record. (If 1:59 is someday recorded at Boston, so be it.)

Those of us who run in marathons usually think of time as a factor that continuously works *against* us, and it certainly can have that psychological effect. But as history has clearly shown, there is no running event in which the times don't go faster. Whether it's 100 meters or 26.2 miles, records will continue to be broken. This reflects an inevitability that's deeply rooted inside human nature. We thrive on competition and the ceaseless need to outshine the past. We want to stand apart from our rivals by being the best at something. Once a runner finally makes it to 1:59, expect to see other runners immediately rise to the challenge and attempt to go even faster.

THE MILE

The marathon is comprised of 26.2 miles, but it's the sole running event in the Olympics that is non-metric. Moreover, metric distances continue to dominate the international racing scene. The stand-alone mile long ago lost its luster as one of the gold standards for distance running. Since 1976, the mile is the only non-metric distance recognized by the International Association of Athletics Federations (IAAF) for record purposes.

Yet training and racing for a marathon is learning how to smartly and efficiently string together twenty-six individual one-mile blocks (and the final 385 yards). That is why the mile continues to hold such a strong emotional and physical attachment with almost all runners. The distance acts as our training and racing baseline, whether we log miles on the track, treadmill, or road. To reach 1:59 flat, a runner will need to click off a mind-staggering succession of 4:33-mile splits.

Mile is derived from the Latin or Roman word *mille*, or 1,000, because a mile was the distance a Roman legion could typically march in 1,000 paces (or 2,000 steps, with the pace being the distance between successive falls of the same foot). Roman soldiers were quite fast marchers. They typically covered twenty-five miles in five hours while carrying a seventy-pound backpack and wearing their body armor.

For centuries following the fall of the Roman Empire, miles of varying lengths were used throughout Western Europe. In 1592, the British Parliament finally settled the question by defining the statute mile to be 8 furlongs, 80 chains, 320 rods, 1,760 yards or 5,280 feet.

The mile then began to be used in different ways, not just to calculate distances between towns, but in sporting events known as pedestrianism. In the middle and late 1800s, race walking on oval tracks was a popular spectator sport in England and the US. The very best walkers could cover 100 miles within 24 hours. Sometimes, these races lasted for six days. Gambling helped fuel their growth as a sport, but pedestrianism died out when it was discovered that many of the competitions were fixed.

In 1886, Englishman Walter George clocked 4:12 as the first official mile record. It is also the same time that Svetlana Masterkova, of Russia, established as the women's mile-world record 110 years later in 1996.

Throughout the 1930s and 1940s (except during the Second World War), the mile remained one of the marquee events in track and field. In 1945, the mile record stood at 4:01.4, and was set by the Swedish runner Gunder Haag. And for nine years, the record went untouched. Many track experts believed that humans simply couldn't run any faster, and that it was absurd to think that someone could run a mile under four minutes.

But British medical student Roger Bannister thought otherwise. He had additional motivation following a disappointing 1952 Stockholm Olympics in which he failed to medal. For nearly two years, he trained exclusively for the mile. When he laced up his kangaroo-leather track shoes with extra-long spikes on May 6, 1954, he believed that he was ready to make history on that cinder-ash track in Oxford, England. All he needed to do was whittle away 4/10ths of a second for each lap, or 1.5 seconds overall.

Bannister ran that celebrated mile even faster, in 3 minutes and 59.4 seconds. His two pacesetters had positioned him well for a 59-second final lap. By his own estimation, Bannister said afterwards that he had run 20,000 miles in eight years of ceaseless preparation for the day of reckoning.

Seven weeks later, Australian John Landy broke Bannister's record by going 3:58. Earlier, Landy had said the following after running a 4:02 mile: "Frankly, I think the four-minute mile is beyond my capabilities. Two seconds may not sound much, but to me it's like trying to break through a brick wall."

The times for the mile have continued to drop since 1954. Runners have set world records from a variety of countries—Ireland, New Zealand, United States, England, France, Algeria, Morocco, Sweden, and Tanzania. But oddly, no Kenyans or Ethiopians appear on this list. Hicham El Guerrouj, of Morocco, currently holds the world record in 3:43.13. The fastest mile ever run by an American belongs to Alan Webb, in 3:46.91.

Bannister, arguably the most famous miler in history, is also the one who held the world record for the shortest period of time.

Surprisingly, it took years after Bannister ran that mile before anyone seriously challenged the notion that it was physiologically possible to run *two* sub-4 minute miles back-to-back. Yet, in 1997, Kenya's Daniel Komen ran two miles in less than eight minutes (7:58.61), setting a world record. No one has since equaled Komen's feat.

CHAPTER 2

K-FACTOR

It's the road signs, "Beware of lions."

—BERNARD LAGAT, bronze medalist in 1,500 meters at
the 2004 Sydney Olympics, explaining why his country
of Kenya produces so many great runners

Will our 1:59 marathoner be a Kenyan? Based on today's fastest marathon times, there's a strong probability that a runner from that country will be the barrier-breaker. The four fastest marathoners in 2013 were all Kenyans, with a range of 2:03:23–2:04:05. The Kenyans consistently win the big marathons. They do it in fluid, red-black-green lockstep style. The first five finishers at the 2013 Berlin Marathon, were all Kenyans. At the 2013 Chicago Marathon, the top four runners were also Kenyans. They now regularly win at New York City and Tokyo. While a Kenyan did not win the 2014 Boston Marathon (that honor went to Meb Keflezighi, who was born in Eritrea and immigrated to the United States as a child), this nation of distance runners had won 19 of the last 23 races. The only other country that regularly breaks Kenya's 26.2-mile chokehold is its neighbor to the north, Ethiopia. It just so happens that the next five fastest marathon times of 2013 belong to Ethiopian runners.

East Africa is home to a majority of the world's fastest marathoners. But as I will later show in this chapter, its domination in distance running won't continue indefinitely. In fact, runners from other countries might soon replace the Wilsons, Emmanuels, Dennises, Sammys, Eliuds, and Tsegayes, who come from Kenya and Ethiopia.

Both nations have a rich, proud, and historical tradition when it comes to distance running. Their long-distance runners now make up more than 90 percent of the all-time world records. As countries without the distraction of major professional sports like basketball, baseball, or football, their national pastime is running. Top runners are treated as wealthy celebrities, heroes to children and adults.

Kenya and Ethiopia share many similarities—high-altitude, a predominantly rural culture built around hard manual labor, children going barefoot and running to school almost every day, the presence of local running clubs and cross-country races, an emphasis on rigorous training accompanied by easy recovery runs, and the widespread recognition that running offers one of the only means to escape poverty. For example, the average annual wage in Kenya is $1,700, but a professional runner can bank well over $100,000 by winning a race like the Chicago Marathon, and even a lot more with performance bonuses, appearance fees, and a lucrative shoe deal.

Understandably, exercise researchers and running journalists are fascinated by Kenya. Their focus centers on the small town of Iten, which is about 210 miles northwest of the capital, Nairobi. Perched at 8,000 feet in the Upper Rift Valley, this town of 4,000 attracts not just professional Kenyan runners, but also distinguished distance runners from all over the world. In Iten, one finds international teams, marathon winners, Olympic medalists (including Stephen Kiprotich, an Ugandan who won marathon gold in the 2012 London Games in 2:08:01 under hot, sunny, and humid conditions), and hundreds more who eke out a decent living by doing well in low-profile races.

On a typical early morning in Iten, you might see numerous packs of runners, often fending off the chill in brightly colored running suits, getting in their first workout of the day, moving along in a dazzling blur on the surrounding dirt roads and hilly trails. Iten also supports ancillary businesses—training camps, sports tourism, coaches, agents, cooks, and physical trainers. It is a one-industry town, and that industry just happens to be running. It is not uncommon to find up to 100 runners temporarily living at the popular High Altitude Training Centre.

The village of Bekoji in Ethiopia's highlands also attracts outside runners from the West as well as ongoing media interest, because it has produced an amazing number of champion long-distance runners who have won 16 Olympic medals in the past two decades.

In 2011, Reid Coolsaet, whose marathon PR of 2:10:55 is the third fastest ever run by a Canadian, spent one month in Iten, hoping to learn firsthand from the Kenyans. Writing in Toronto's *Globe and Mail* newspaper, Coolsaet discussed what it was like to live and train in this cradle of distance running:

Kenyans are no exception when it comes to logging many kilometers day in, day out. Most of the runners I met run at least twice a day but some run up to three times. After bouts of hard training it is vital that the body has time to repair and recover for the next training session. Kenyan runners incorporate naps into their days and get to bed early. Plus, they don't run hard all the time; most people would be surprised on how slow they run their recovery runs.

When I was in Iten, all of my running was on trails and dirt roads (of course, this is easy to do when there is only one paved road in the area). Seeing a Kenyan run alone is the exception to the norm. Kenyans run in groups during speed sessions as well as their easy runs. Many times while I was running with Kenyans I was surprised how slowly they would start off.

If you are an elite Kenyan runner, in which running is pretty much all you do and have known your entire life, then training with your equally talented peers offers a uniquely competitive advantage. Geoffrey Mutai, who ran 2:03:02 at the 2011 Boston Marathon, has two regular training partners: world marathon-record holder, Wilson Kipsang, and Dennis Kimetto, who won the Chicago Marathon in a course-record time of 2:03:45.

In a 2013 interview with a Kenyan radio station, Mutai chocked up his success to the following: "It is all about training harder and harder in these hills and valleys that are in places like here or Iten, staying focused and when you make it, avoiding the kind of lifestyle that will finish your strength."

Besides all that focused training in Iten, what else has contributed to Kenya's dominance in distance running? Many seek an explanation for the country's success by looking at human biology. One of the most tossed-about questions by the media is this: Are Kenyans genetically superior to distance runners from other non-East African countries?

Personally, I don't think the answer can be found in their DNA, because after a decade of advanced genetic research, scientists have still been unable to locate any specific genetic markers indicating endurance superiority in Kenyan runners.

Instead, I'd like to argue that endurance ability is determined by personal and environmental factors—how one trains, where one lives, amount of rest and recovery, nutrition, and mental outlook. Sure, most elite Kenyan runners are small-stature, lean, and have whippet-thin legs, so they aren't carrying extra weight, but equally important is living at high altitude, spending most of one's early years active and barefoot, and coming from a place where running is a national sport.

The problem with wanting to attribute Kenya's success to a single variable—"the endurance gene"—is not only bad science but that it totally ignores much more relevant training and lifestyle considerations. Those who make the claim that Kenya's supremacy in distance running has to do with genes are often speaking from relative ignorance about the highly complex field of genetics. At the same time, if a scientist's published research suggests the presence of a strong, empirical connection between race and natural athletic ability, the critical reaction is usually hostile. Even writing about race and athletics in the media, or bringing up the sensitive topic if you are a sports broadcaster, is apparently taboo.

IS THE DOOR CLOSING ON KENYA'S SUPREMACY?

Runners from other nations and cultures have dominated distance running since the early 1900s. The United States' first wave of great runners were American Indians, and the swiftest came from the Hopi Tribe, who had a deeply spiritual reverence for running as a means to connect to their ancestors and gods. The most famous Hopi runner, Lewis Tewanima, twice represented the US in the Olympics and picked up the silver in the 10,000 meters at the 1912 Stockholm Games. Fifty-two years passed before another American medaled in the 10,000 meters, when Billy Mills, who was of Sioux descent, took gold.

Finland ruled the middle- and long-distance international scene for several decades, beginning with the 1912 Olympics. Its runners were known as "The Flying Finns." Years later, at the 1972 Munich Olympics and 1976 Montreal Games, the last of the great Flying

Finns, Lasse Viren, won a total of four golds in the 5,000 meters and 10,000 meters.

After the Second World War, England was a powerhouse in middle-distance running (the mile, not the marathon, was the crowd-drawing attraction). Then along came other English-speaking nations—New Zealand, Australia, and Ireland—which produced a number of world-record milers and middle-distance champions. The US wasn't far behind, led by world-class miler Jim Ryun, who became the first high-school runner to break four minutes for the mile, going 3:59.0 as a junior. This period lasted for little more than a decade right up until the late 1970s. Frank Shorter's marathon victory in the 1972 Munich Olympics is widely viewed as the catalyst for running's first boom in America. Ever since, it's been the Africans who have established themselves as the world's best—from the North (primarily the Moroccans and Algerians) and the East (Kenyans, Ethiopians, and to a lesser degree, Eritreans). In recent years, Kenya has pulled away from the pack of its fellow East African contenders.

How long will Kenya remain on top? Is the door closing on Kenya's supremacy? And if so, why? Will we someday see another nation, besides Ethiopia, become home to the fastest distance runners? And if so, which nation or nations?

There are at least two important factors that lead me to believe that Kenya will one day see its dominance begin to falter. It probably won't happen overnight, and might take a generation or two of runners for this change to become most apparent. The first factor has to do with genetics; the other is environmental. Both have been touted as the reasons for success in the endurance world. They are also deeply intertwined, and affect each other in profound ways. This relationship can be distilled as nature/nurture.

- Nature is our natural-born biology, with genes that provide the blueprint of being human. We pass on this genetic material from one generation to the next in the form of DNA, which contains codes that dictate specific features that the newborn will possess. As examples, these include hair and eye color, body height, basic body build, and skin color. It has taken millions of years of natural selection for our genes to become what they are today.

- Nurture is the environment's effect on our body. This includes diet, stress, lifestyle and one's upbringing. In particular, the development of physical activity in early childhood can significantly influence one's ability to run faster or slower later in life.

The web of nature and nurture interactions is intricate and detailed. Diet and physical activity can turn on—or off—specific genes. So if genes dictate a person will have an adult height of five feet six inches, poor nutrition may diminish that—the most common example is a child who is protein-malnourished and does not attain normal height.

While some genes clearly contribute to running ability, including those affecting enzymes that are associated with aerobic metabolism, there is no guarantee that they will be naturally turned on. Nor are these genes so powerful or unique to any one population of humans, or even a particular geographical area.

The genes can't magically transform the human body into an accomplished marathoner. If a marathon gene did in fact exist, such as one that determines eye color, there would be many more magnificent Kenyan and Ethiopian runners. But instead, for every elite East African marathoner already running in the 2:03–2:08 range, there are hundreds of others who might have tried just as hard but somehow didn't make the superior grade and become star runners.

One of the key factors associated with superb endurance is the combined importance of VO_2max, lactate threshold, and running economy in achieving optimal marathon performance. Specifically, how well do the Kenyans fare in these areas?

Human endurance expert Dr. Michael Joyner has written that "a careful review of the scientific studies shows that [the Kenyans'] values are nothing special for elite distance runners. However, many do have outstanding values for running economy, but these values are not better than those seen in the most efficient whites. Also, no genetic factors have been identified to explain their success." Joyner does state that if the East Africans have something unique, "It is likely due to hard and active lives at high altitude from an early age."

The environment also has a direct influence on genes. An example is skin color, which is genetically determined. The evolution of the full spectrum of skin—from the darkest to the lightest—is due to the pigment *melanin*, which is stimulated by sunlight. As the earliest humans, who were dark-skinned, migrated away from the equator and eventually out of Africa, they encountered reduced sunlight in the more northern and southern regions of the world; over many generations, their skin color gradually lightened. The greater the distance from the equator these populations lived, the lighter, and whiter their skin became.

Skin color is related to another important nature/nurture issue, and it's one that points to why the East Africans may not continue their endurance-running dominance. This has to do with the steady exodus to the West by their young, promising runners, barely out of their teens, who are seeking a better life in the US and Europe. Living near the equator's strong sun means better vitamin D status for those with dark skin. This is especially true at higher altitudes, where there is less sun-blocking moisture in the air. But for a Kenyan runner who spends most of the year racing and traveling to cities with significantly less sun exposure, this can lead to insufficient vitamin D.

An additional environmental hazard is the temptation of an unhealthy diet that's so common in the West. Even lean runners are not spared sudden weight gain. Bad, junk food eating (and a resulting increase in body fat) can be triggered by the stress of too much racing and living in a foreign country. To make matters worse, the regular consumption of all those refined carbohydrates is a double-edged sword when it comes to genetics. First, these harmful carbs can turn on genes that cause diseases such as diabetes. Second, by replacing nutrient-rich healthy foods in the diet, the lack of good nutrients that would normally trigger healthy gene effects are now absent. This can also lead to poor health and symptoms such as asthma, fatigue, and even physical injuries.

For Kenyan runners who are in their racing prime, it's truly a race against time. The more successful they are as marathoners, the greater becomes the likelihood that they will spend more time in the West where serious environmental pitfalls can and do exist. And then, within a few years or even less, there is the potential of a noticeable decline in performance. Unfortunately, this falling off can occur long before a runner reaches his best years—something we already see in many of today's great marathoners. Burnout is a real problem. Plus, there's always other runners back home in Kenya who are ready and eager to race professionally in the West. For runners who are at the early stage of their racing careers, this kind of competitive pressure can contribute to intense emotional and mental stress, leading to poor training and racing decisions. The Kenyan Moses Tanui, who won the Boston Marathon in 1996 and 1998, said it best: "Kenyan runners don't retire; they simply disappear."

VITAMIN D

The high-altitude environment in Kenya allows runners to train all year round under a strong sun. This exposure promotes the production of vitamin D despite dark skin. More than adequate levels are essential for optimal training and racing, and not enough is available from foods. This nutrient is critical for brain, bone, and muscle health, not to mention controlling inflammation, preventing injuries, reducing muscle fatigue, and improving performance. Athletes with vitamin D deficiencies may also have smaller hearts.

Unfortunately, not enough studies have been done on runners' vitamin D status or levels. In a recent study presented at the 2011 annual meeting of the American Orthopedic Society for Sports Medicine, vitamin D levels were tested in eighty-nine professional football players. Only twenty had bare-minimal levels with 80 percent being vitamin D deficient. Lead researcher Dr. Michael Shindle said that, "African-American players and players who suffered muscle injuries had significantly lower levels." Overall, mean vitamin levels in whites were 30 (ng/mL) and only 20 in blacks.

Those of us who have worked with international athletes of all races have found essentially the same pattern—those with darker skin usually have the lowest vitamin D levels. I should emphasize that the exception is the athlete who remains in his or her natural environment much of the time. That's why Kenyan runners migrating to foreign lands with less sun exposure risk the problem of reduced vitamin D and impaired endurance ability. This is especially the case as athletes age into their later twenties and early and mid-thirties—the period when marathon performance should peak.

In addition to skin color, sunscreen use (which blocks vitamin D production), avoidance of sun (training early or late in the day), and air pollution (which blocks sunlight) can significantly lower the sun's ability to raise vitamin D levels. And, this pro-hormone vitamin plays a key role in turning on healthy genes—or turning them off when levels are inadequate.

In addition, a recent study appearing in the *American Journal of Clinical Nutrition* shows that African Americans require a higher vitamin D dose to maintain healthy levels compared to those with white skin.

This problem has a remedy. Short of staying in one's natural environment much of the time, a simple dietary supplement of vitamin D-containing fish liver oil could help correct deficiencies of this nutrient and maintain healthy levels. However, that is easier said than done in some cases. It requires regular testing, and assessing other nutrients and body fat content, all of which can affect vitamin D status.

The potential downside for vitamin D supplementation is that, in too high a dose, it can be toxic and significantly impair health.

Despite their deep bench of blazing-fast marathoners, the Kenyans and perhaps the Ethiopians won't always continue to be so invincible. Today's winners don't always stay on top. They get beaten. They lose. Others surpass them. I can't indicate when this might occur, but a possible turning point could become first evident at a major marathon, when, despite a packed field of East Africans, few make the top ten.

Of course, it is certainly possible that the process has already started. Today, there are far too many Kenyans and Ethiopians who have begun their decline long before their bodies should have started failing them (something I further detail in Appendix B). The accumulated impact of travel, poor diet, and nutrient imbalance can often lead to injury, reduced health, and poor performance.

In an interview with the British edition of *Runner's World,* Moses Tanui, who was also the first man to ever run a half-marathon under 60 minutes, provided this singular perspective on the current state of affairs affecting his countrymen:

You compete with yourself and the course when you run a marathon. I trained for endurance and speed. I ran seven days a week, twice a day—sometimes three times. I ran 300 kilometers a week . . . Kenyan runners all want to do the marathon these days because there's so much money to be made. A Kenyan man might win one marathon and never win another because he's too young to have built a strong endurance base and he doesn't know how to recover properly.

Moreover, the window of opportunity to run 1:59 might even be in jeopardy of closing for the East Africans. Should their dominance begin to wane, who will become the next generation of great distance runners? Will we see an explosion of marathon talent from South Africa, which already has a strong running tradition, as anyone who has been to the Comrades race can attest? Should we look to Asia? Will it be runners from Japan that is gripped with marathon mania, and whose professional runners are just a step behind the East Africans in several of the big marathons? Can South Korea rise to the challenge? Or is China the sleeping marathon giant?

Finally, can the US keep up, or will it continue to fade into endurance obscurity? No doubt, American runners are extremely talented. But instead of the occasional athlete excelling in the marathon, half-marathon, or 10,000 meters, many more elite runners need to avoid the "no pain, no gain" training mindset that starts in grade school and continues right through college and beyond. (And spending more time barefoot while growing up will help.) Runners in the US must learn to adopt a balanced, healthy athletic lifestyle. Until this important change or reawakening occurs, top American runners will continue to suffer from an epidemic of training-related injuries. While it is entirely likely that an American will someday make it to 1:59, how many runners from other countries will have gotten there first?

CHAPTER 3
RUNNING ECONOMY

I was just lucky in terms of the biomechanics.

—BILL RODGERS

The lead runners in a big-city marathon are fun to watch. They relentlessly push forward with natural ease, a testament to their athletic gifts. Their lean bodies seem perfectly suited to running— torso slightly facing forward, head held straight, legs powering off their midfoot. These runners have what is called excellent running economy. But runners lagging behind the leaders most likely have reduced running economy. They often appear to be struggling.

Then, compare these elite marathoners with the rest of the field, which often numbers in the thousands or more, and the differences are much more apparent. A significant number of these runners have poor, inefficient physical form as their bodies are unable to maximize their energy potential. In fact, they are wasting energy. These runners are much more likely to experience fatigue long before they reach the finish line. Many end up walking.

Here's another way to view the importance of running economy. Humans prefer taking the course of least resistance. We want quick results, whether it's trying to lose weight, get in shape, make money, or complete a marathon. In many ways, it is more difficult to run a marathon in 4:05 than in 2:05. Those extra two hours on the course require increased oxygen, additional muscle contraction, and are accompanied by greater wear and tear on the body. The goal of improving running economy is to make the marathon easier on the body.

Running economy (RE) is sometimes referred to as running efficiency. Optimal RE is absolutely essential for a 1:59 marathon.

Running economy is usually evaluated on a treadmill while measuring oxygen utilization. Going at the same pace, a runner with better economy will use less oxygen than one whose economy is subpar. While RE can be expressed in terms of oxygen use, it's more accurate to examine energy needs. The more economical one's running becomes the less energy is needed in the forms of burning body fat and sugar.

Improvement in one's RE can result in six positive outcomes:
- As training progresses, one can run faster at the same submaximal heart rate.
- There is an increased utilization of body fat for fuel.
- There is a preservation of glycogen stores during training and racing.
- Race pace quickens.
- Recovery from training and racing is more rapid.
- Reduction, if not elimination, of injuries and illness.

Improvements in RE can be measured with a heart rate monitor. (This is detailed in the next chapter.) Unfortunately, exercise scientists have not measured large enough numbers of elite runners to gather sufficient information about RE. Yet here are two specific examples of runners who reportedly improved their RE on their way to accomplishing world records:

- Steve Scott broke the American record for the mile in 1982. Exercise physiologist Gary Krahenbuhl says that over a period of eighteen weeks, Scott improved his RE by 5 percent.
- In 2003, England's Paula Radcliffe set the marathon world record of 2:15. Previous to that, her RE increased 14 percent over a five-year period, which equated to running 40 seconds per mile faster without changing how much oxygen she took in.

IMPROVING RE

One of the most important ways to improve RE is training the body's aerobic muscle fibers—which are also referred to as slow-twitch (or type 1)—and by spending less time performing traditional track intervals, weights, and anaerobic workouts. In the textbook *Essentials of Exercise Physiology* (2006, third edition), the coauthors, Drs. William McArdle, Frank Katch, and Victor Katch, state a well-accepted but often forgotten fact about training: "Activation of slow-twitch fibers produces greater efficiency than the same work accomplished by fast-twitch fibers." Aerobic muscles are essentially more economical, and burn fat as fuel. This is particularly true for marathon training.

The concept of training slow-twitch muscle fibers is neither new nor radical. It's been around for decades. Many of the first marathoners and other distance runners eventually discovered that training slower was more natural and equally effective than trying to run hard all the time. In the 1950s and 1960s, two running coaches emphasized longer, slower marathon training. German physician Ernst van Aaken helped bring the concept of long slow distance (LSD) to endurance training. Famed New Zealand coach Arthur Lydiard successfully emphasized slow-twitch training for aerobic-base work.

When I started coaching runners in the 1970s, I made every effort to emphasize aerobic training and its correlation with increased fat burning. Many of these runners initially felt uncomfortable running at slower speeds. But over time, they found that they were running just as fast as before (or even faster) but at a lower heart rate because they were becoming more economical.

So why is there such a continued emphasis on fierce, lung-busting anaerobic workouts? More specifically, do track-interval sessions offer substantial benefits for distance runners? As running became more popular in the 1970s, the sport attracted coaches—many of whom crossed over from track-and-field. They brought with them their successful work ethic: intervals. This approach is most effective when training for events up to 10,000 meters. But the marathon is very different. A 10K or shorter race is a highly anaerobic event, requiring near VO_2max. But competing over 26.2 miles is successfully accomplished around 85 percent of one's VO_2max. For energy needs in the longer race, it's stored body fat that provides the much-needed fuel.

Tapping into the energy reserves of body fat—which fuels the aerobic muscle fibers—will be necessary for a 1:59 marathon because it offers an unlimited supply. But if the use of fat for fuel is limited, or the aerobic fibers are undertrained, then more sugar must fuel the muscles. This not only limits one's energy, but also reduces RE. Maintaining stable blood-sugar levels and avoiding glycogen depletion is vital during a marathon, even for one lasting 1:59, and helps maintain fat burning, and good RE.

Almost all types of training—including hard efforts—can increase VO_2max and lactate threshold, even during overtraining in its early stages. But this won't necessarily improve performance because running economy may actually diminish. Unfortunately, what often happens is that runners try to push their VO_2max and lactate thresholds higher at the *expense* of RE. The net result is usually diminished performance.

However, by increasing the function of the aerobic muscle fibers and related body components—the heart, lungs, circulation, and fat burning, each part of what I call the aerobic system—RE can improve significantly. This is indicated by faster training at the same heart rate, leading to a swifter race pace. The well-developed aerobic system is an untapped source of performance potential. It can greatly boost RE.

Here's a condensed summary of other factors that impact RE. They are applicable for all runners, no matter one's age, natural ability, or racing experience. Please note: these factors are subsequently discussed in much greater detail in forthcoming chapters.

Overreaching. The sweet spot of training means enough volume (time/miles) but not too much, and going fast but not too fast. This point is called overreaching, which more than maintains fitness, but is before the onset of overtraining. To properly arrive at this sweet spot, here's my high-performance formula: Training = Workout + Rest.

Muscle Balance. Even a slight irregularity in the gait can reduce running economy. The neuromuscular system—the brain and muscles—regulates one's movements. But if muscle imbalance develops, gait problems follow. This may be associated with poor footwear, unhealthy diet, or overtraining. A separate muscle issue is strength—a surprising number of runners don't have enough. But traditional weight-lifting routines can often impair aerobic function, increase muscle fatigue, and reduce endurance, all leading to sub-par running economy.

The Feet. Our feet (and lower legs) allow us to harness the gravitational impact forces from hitting the ground, turning that contact into additional energy. This unique energy-return system can be significant. But it won't work well in feet that are dysfunctional, leading to lost economy. Extra energy is robbed by muscle imbalance, overstretched tendons, inflexibility, and associated problems due to poor foot function that are related to wearing bad shoes. You want to avoid rigid, over-supported running shoes that have thick soles and outsized heels. Many chronic foot problems can be minimized by finding the ideal shoe for each foot, or eliminated entirely by running barefoot.

Healthy Foods. The foods we eat can directly affect RE by enhancing fat burning, balancing muscles, increasing circulation, controlling free radicals and helping to build a better aerobic body. The most serious barrier to fat burning and endurance potential is refined carbohydrates—stay clear of them if you want to improve running economy.

Altitude. For decades, endurance athletes have sought altitude training as a way to get faster. But this is misleading. *Living* at higher elevations, such as 7,000–8,000 feet, can help improve running economy, while training at lower elevations, 4,000 feet or below, is best. However, just going to altitude does not guarantee results. That's because the process first requires a healthy body. A poor diet, for example, may not supply all the nutritional needs, such as iron, folic acid, or protein, necessary for altitude living to increase quality red blood cells and better aerobic function.

The Brain. It's the brain that improves the body's running economy. While the brain is the most misunderstood and most neglected part of an athlete, it regulates, directly or indirectly, all the factors noted above.

WEAKENING RE

Many runners think they can become faster by copying the form of an elite athlete. They do all they can to mimic this "perfect" gait. They may even employ various training techniques or watch instructional videos to learn how to consciously move isolated body parts, seeking to replicate what essentially can't be reproduced. It's tempting to envision that by just elevating the knees slightly more, or swinging the arms like so, one will become the runner that is the stuff of dreams. But a one-size-fits-all approach doesn't guarantee the likelihood of good running economy, and as is often the case, this can actually worsen it.

There's also the mistaken assumption that training itself will improve RE. In fact, some of the more common approaches employed

RUNNING ECONOMY TAKE AWAY

Here are several RE guidelines: Try running relaxed and natural, and do not think about emulating someone else's style. Almost all runners tend to automatically find their most efficient gaits. This occurs because the brain figures out how to be most economical;

it works with the body, *not* against it. Then, by improving specific body functions—the feet, aerobic system, and diet—the brain can create the most efficient movements leading to an improvement of RE.

in preparing for a marathon often reduce running economy due to excess wear and tear, overtraining, inadequate rest and recovery, and reduced emphasis on aerobic function.

THE 1:45 MARATHON?

Significant improvements in RE could even lower marathon times far below the holy grail of 1:59. In an article entitled "Endurance Exercise Performance: The Physiology of Champions," which was published in 2007 in the *Journal of Physiology*, Dr. Michael Joyner argued that the human body is physiologically capable of running a 1:45 marathon—nearly twelve minutes faster than his 1991 estimates in the same journal! By using the common equation used to predict marathon times—*VO₂max x Lactate threshold percentage x Running efficiency*—he showed that when reasonable estimates of the best values ever recorded for these three parameters are tabulated, the fastest possible marathon approached 1:45. Joyner states, "Even when assumptions about wind resistance were added, times well under 2 hours seemed possible."

Using the same data and including information about muscle balance and fat burning, I calculated the potential of today's top marathoners. Based on greatly improving these runners' RE—exercise scientists have estimated that this can vary dramatically by a staggering 20 to 30 percent—I believe that a 1:48 marathon is within the realm of possibility. While I am not as generous as Joyner, what's three minutes when we are this far south of 1:59? Another way to consider the potential likelihood of a sub-1:50 marathon is that a 1:59 time is actually a conservative prediction of where several world-class runners should be at now.

Running economy incorporates, at least in the ideal sense, all the functions of body and brain. We may never know how important any one component may be. But we do know that a range of factors, including muscles, lungs, heart, and brain must work in harmony to run a fast marathon. In addition, while VO_2max and lactate threshold diminish with age, RE does not always follow in pursuit—the reason our 1:59 marathoner may be in his thirties.

Running economy should be looked at holistically. This means that factors such as aerobic function, blood-sugar regulation, circulation, breathing, and red-blood cell function can specifically influence RE. Good, overall health is critical for optimal RE. A 1:59 marathon can be run relatively soon, and will require a significant improvement in running economy. Monitoring the body every step of the way can help individualize one's training and lifestyle. The guesswork is eliminated. The importance of testing the body and individualization is the topic of the next chapter.

CHAPTER 4

RUNNER OF ONE

Know why people run marathons? Because running is rooted in our collective imagination, and our imagination is rooted in running. Language, art, science; space shuttles, Starry Night*, intravascular surgery; they all had their roots in our ability to run. Running was the superpower that made us human.*

—CHRISTOPHER MCDOUGALL, author of *Born to Run*

No two runners are alike. Each runner is unique, a true individual. In order to pull off 1:59, our marathoner must learn how to drown out the noise of bad information, tradition, and misguided advice from well-meaning coaching experts. Yes, he must run by feel, relying on instinct and intuition, because the brain is a mighty impressive pilot. But in today's world of hype and misrepresentation, runners are heavily influenced by the media that love to oversimplify things, by advertisements, and by the generalized cookbook approach to training.

That is why a 1:59 marathon will only become a reality if the runner monitors every step of training through the objective process of evaluation, or what is also called assessment. In the course of regular testing, a runner benefits from the confidence-enhancing knowledge that real progress is being made, instead of waiting for the first sign of an injury or doubts about performance. Assessment may appear a bit tedious to implement, especially at first, but its application can separate a winner from those finishing just steps behind him.

The late Dr. George Sheehan, who was a colleague, friend, lecturer, and best-selling author, helped influence and inspire many Americans to take up running in the 1970s and 1980s. An excellent age-group athlete who began participating in marathons rather late in life, George, who ran track in college, frequently brought up the concept of individualization, or what he referred to as an "experiment of one." Each runner must find out what works best for himself or herself. It's only by trial-and-error that a runner can maximize athletic potential. But the goal of objective assessment is to speed up the learning process, to eliminate preventable mistakes that can be made along the way. Assessment effectively identifies those potential obstacles that usually impair optimal performance in both training and racing.

Our 1:59 runner will have to make adjustments based on measurable assessments. These changes could be minor (or possibly, major) alterations in diet, lifestyle, training, or recovery. He will also be an "experiment of one." Or more accurately, he's an "experiment of one fifty-nine."

Almost every runner who has been in the sport for some time has encountered a plateau—which can seem more like a brick wall of frustration—when training and racing times appear to have stalled or begin to show evidence of a gradual decline. This scenario often creates intense bouts of anxiety, especially if there aren't any outward signs of a physical injury, even a slight one. In a futile effort to reverse matters, many runners begin to train ever harder. Yet this approach seldom works because there are often several factors affecting performance. Silent-harm culprits can be such things as stress, lack of sleep (even an hour less every 24 hours makes a big difference), or an unhealthy diet.

Professional runners are unlike most recreational athletes, in large part due to the year-round pressure of travel and racing. One's career must navigate that tricky divide separating injury or poor health and the desire to train harder, race faster, and win more often.

For those few runners who have successfully made it inside the exclusive 2:03–2:05 zone, there's even greater pressure to keep pushing and hopefully get to 2:02, and subsequently lower. At this elite level, the hunger to race faster and set a new record can easily morph into a maddening quest. The two-hour marathon is unlike any other barrier in the athletic world. Breaking it is both achingly close and deceptively out of reach. Whoever gets there first will make instant history. *But in order to become the Roger Bannister of marathon, our record-setting 1:59 runner must first adopt assessment as a key element to his training regimen.* Running simply by feel is insufficient.

It is difficult for most runners to be objective about their own bodies. Even trained health professionals who are experts at making sense of abnormal signs and symptoms sometimes find it difficult when assessing patients. Nonetheless, piecing together these clues from a runner's body is potentially the difference between progress and regress, success and failure. There can be a slight niggle in the knee, a peculiar twinge in the foot, the onset of afternoon fatigue, or a change in appetite. Any of these symptoms can be meaningful indicators because they may directly relate to an oncoming problem.

Race performance is the most popular method to gauge a runner's success. Consistently poor race times are a more obvious indication of a potentially debilitating problem. Just the opposite is true for terrific results. But for a marathoner, who does not race that distance often enough to gather adequate data within a sufficient period, improved performance can sometimes be misleading. The results of a race or two can actually be deceptive. A common example is a runner who, in the early stage of overtraining, might pull off a PR (but by minutes, not seconds). This occurs because the sympathetic nervous system is overactive and stress hormones are high, leading to a temporary performance enhancement. If adequate recovery does not offset the overtraining, the situation can later lead to a sudden decline in performance, the onset of a physical injury, or a chemical one such as fatigue.

Rather than risk being fooled into thinking all is going fine, runners should engage in ongoing, proper assessments during regular training—think of these measurements as personal evaluations. They can provide important objective information about progress.

One of the more popular assessments is a runner's maximum oxygen uptake, which is called VO_2max. Another way to describe VO_2max is how efficiently your muscles utilize oxygen during maximum effort. Scientifically, it is measured as milliliters of oxygen used in one minute per kilogram of body weight. The theory goes that the more oxygen you can use during a high-level exercise, the more ATP (adenosine triphosphate) energy your body can produce. Endurance athletes, and not just marathoners, but cyclists, swimmers, and cross-country skiers, have very high VO_2max values compared to the general population. For example, an untrained male's VO_2max may be 45, while an elite marathoner is above 75.

Traditionally, VO_2max is often said to be the so-called gold standard in athletic assessment. However, others believe it is a highly overrated test. Why is that the case? There are several reasons.

First, it's misleading to think that elite athletes frequently undergo complicated laboratory measurements, usually wired up on a treadmill, while breathing through a tube and running at top speed. But many prefer to avoid these evaluations with any regularity. While some of these laboratory tests certainly have potentially significant value—and I have performed many of them—the test is performed on a treadmill in a lab. So it is not an accurate representation of a runner out on the road or track. Endurance expert Dr. Michael Joyner writes that "VO_2max is a good predictor of performance if you test a very large number of people with a wide range of values. However, it does not mean much in a group of elite runners, or any other homogeneous group, or certainly any one individual."

The VO$_2$max test is often done in conjunction with an assessment of lactate threshold, the point when lactate production is greater than its elimination, and it quickly starts to accumulate in the blood. Like with the VO$_2$max, the lactate test assesses anaerobic conditions, and the heart rates related to a runner shifting gears from a maximum aerobic state into an anaerobic one. (At high anaerobic heart rates, muscles produce lactic acid, which goes into the bloodstream and gets converted to lactate.)

For the time being anyway, many exercise physiologists continue to assess VO$_2$max, often relating it to peak performance. Dr. Stephane Delliaux and colleagues at the Faculty of Medicine, Aix-Marseille University, Marseille, France, calculated that former marathon world-record holder Ethiopian Haile Gebrselassie had the "necessary" VO$_2$max of 86 for a 1:59 marathon in the year 2000, at age twenty-seven, when he won all his races and was ranked top in the world in the 5K and 10K. Yet, he ran his best marathon eight years later (2:03:59) when his VO$_2$max would have been on the decline.

The scientific rationale for measuring VO$_2$max has to do with the limitations in performance associated with oxygen flowing through the blood. But more significant than any limitation imposed by oxygen is the brain, which monitors and regulates all the body's physical and biochemical activities. The brain may be the ultimate ceiling in performance, slowing a runner's pace to protect the body from potential serious injury.

South African exercise physiologist Dr. Timothy Noakes, author of the classic *The Lore of Running*, has written extensively about the myths of VO$_2$max testing. In a 2008 article, "Testing for Maximum

Oxygen Consumption has Produced a Brainless Model of Human Exercise Performance," which appeared in the *British Journal of Sports Medicine,* Noakes wrote that many people in sport "are apparently wedded to the concept that oxygen delivery alone determines the power output of the exercising limbs, and thus, they appear blind to a converse interpretation." Noakes believes that the development of the VO_2max test probably explains why most people in sports seldom consider that the brain's effect on muscle function could be an important regulator of athletic performance.

Despite these reservations about its efficacy, VO_2max continues to be held in high regard by coaches and their endurance athletes. Both groups like bringing up these personal test numbers in conversation, either with pride or head-scratching frustration ("why isn't it higher?"). It's the same with other test scores such as lactate levels. By themselves, these numbers don't provide enough information to help individualize a marathoner's training, diet, and other lifestyle factors that can significantly influence performance.

What about the current crop of East African distance runners who don't have always the highest VO_2max scores? Dr. Joyner suggests that "the VO_2max values and lactate thresholds for the elite East Africans are impressive but not exceptional for world-class runners." As these runners train into their early- and mid-thirties, performances typically improve while their VO_2max numbers decline.

Elite, older marathon runners often outperform younger runners who have higher VO_2max levels. This is also true for age-groupers. Many male runners have much higher VO_2max levels than female runners, yet a significant number of these women finish ahead of them.

A fast marathon is run at a consistent pace at only around 85 to 88 percent of VO_2max. It will be the same for our 1:59 runner.

Most, if not all, of his pre-race training will take place just below this level, closer to 80 percent of his VO_2max (it may vary depending on the individual). This type of training is the best way to efficiently develop the aerobic system, which allows the body to obtain more energy from fat, conserve glycogen, and avoid the perils of overtraining. (By comparison, racing at distances of 5K and 10K occur close to one's VO_2max, with much of the training at similar levels.)

Great marathons are run at a pace with lactic-acid production just above resting levels rather than higher amounts, and certainly not near one's threshold. But testing lactate levels is more applicable to 5K and 10K distances.

Rather than assessing oxygen utilization on a laboratory treadmill, it is much more important to focus on the two systems of the body—aerobic and anaerobic—and the fuels they generate for race energy.

AEROBIC AND ANAEROBIC

Let's first define the terms aerobic and anaerobic, but in a simple, practical way rather than using complex biochemistry. Basically, aerobic refers to the body's red, slow-twitch muscle fibers, which burn fat for energy. They also rely on sugar to maintain the use of fat for fuel. The aerobic muscles are relied upon for a sub-maximal running pace over various distances. With the right training, one could run quite fast over a long distance at a sub-maximal running pace—even a 5-minute mile pace or faster for over twenty-six miles. (Imagine running 104 consecutive quarter-miles at 75 seconds for each lap.)

The term anaerobic, as discussed here, refers to the use of fast-twitch, sprint-type fibers. Energy is derived from glucose, or sugar burning. The stored form of glucose is glycogen, found in the liver and muscles. While anaerobic is often thought of as being "without oxygen," this designation is misleading and impractical. Certainly there are complex biochemical reactions occurring on a cellular level, but the fact is, runners need to breathe and obtain oxygen all the time—just try holding your breath next time you run at the start of a workout.

Both of these fuels, fat and sugar, generate energy during physical activity (and even rest). The aerobic and anaerobic systems are also working all the time, although the anaerobic actions are usually turned down unless much faster running is necessary, such as for the final kick in a marathon. The aerobic system contributes 99 percent of the energy when racing 26.2 miles.

Let's compare different race distances between the mile and the marathon, in terms of how much energy a runner obtains from the aerobic and anaerobic systems. Below is a chart indicating approximately how much aerobic and anaerobic energy contribution is required to race successfully for a particular runner at various distances. The number of calories (kcal) is also noted in parentheses.

Distance	% Aerobic (kcal)	% Anaerobic (kcal)
Mile	60 (100)	40 (30)
5K	88 (290)	12 (23)
10K	90 (600)	10 (20)
Half Marathon	98 (1200)	2 (15)
Marathon	99 (2600)	1 (5)

Those who burn more stored body fat are generally healthier. For endurance athletes, those using more fat are faster, especially in the marathon. In order to generate adequate amounts of fat, the aerobic system must operate at a high level.

To run a 1:59 marathon, for example, let's say our athlete weighs only 137 pounds. This will require about 2,600 calories of energy from both fat and sugar. A relatively large amount of this energy will come from fat, and the rest from sugar, helping to maintain the process of fat burning.

We don't know the exact mix of fat and sugar that contributes to these total calories as each runner is different. But more success will come to those converting a higher amount of fat stores to energy. Don't be fooled or misled by the low-body fat of elite marathoners. They still rely on converting stored body fat into race energy—even a very lean runner has enough stored fat for many hours of fast running, thanks to a well-developed aerobic system.

If fat burning is impaired or otherwise limited, more sugar will be necessary during a race. This is the case when the aerobic system is not trained extremely well, if a runner goes out too fast (using up too much glycogen in those early miles), or if the pre-race meal contains too many refined carbohydrates, which can diminish fat burning. The result is poor performance due to reduced fat burning and increased reliance on sugar for energy.

Even consuming a sugary sports drink during a race will not make up for a poor aerobic system or reduced fat burning. But those with a great aerobic system that converts large amounts of fat for fuel, a carbohydrate replacement drink may be unnecessary.

In the final kick of the marathon, a runner will rely on more sugar to quicken the pace. Imagine the final several hundred yards with the clock ticking away at 1:58 and change—a fast finish will require a larger amount of available sugar for a burst of speed. If this was not used up during the previous twenty-six miles, there will be enough remaining energy to slip under two hours.

Increasing aerobic function can build the body's fat-burning capability. You can influence the mix of fat and sugar burning through training, diet and other lifestyle factors that minimize stress. All runners can evaluate progress of the aerobic system, and increased fat burning—this is associated with improved running economy and the ability to run faster at the same sub-maximal heart rate (examined in the next chapter). The most accurate assessment of fat and sugar burning can be accomplished in the laboratory, and is discussed below.

RESPIRATORY QUOTIENT

If one ventures into a laboratory, rather than just measuring VO_2max, a similar protocol often performed at the same time can assess how much fat and sugar is used for energy at varying heart rates. This is referred to as the respiratory quotient, or RQ, with a scale ranging from 0.7 (100 percent fat for fuel, zero percent glucose) to 1.0 (zero percent fat and 100 percent glucose for energy). Marathoners have a certain mix of fat and sugar at specific heart rates, and those who burn a higher percentage of fat are faster.

The precise amount of fat that a marathoner burns is individual, depending on the heart rate, how well the aerobic system has been developed, existing stress levels, and the pre-test meal.

The RQ is measured on a treadmill by evaluating the oxygen uptake and carbon dioxide output, and can be correlated with sub-max heart rates and pace. These numbers are a valuable assessment with regular testing because they directly relate to improvements in the aerobic system, and to fat burning.

While RQ can be determined on a treadmill, runners can rely on other important assessments in a more natural environment such as a flat road or track, by measuring their paces at sub-max heart rates. Over weeks and months, an improved pace is associated with building the aerobic system and burning more body fat.

OTHER KEY ASSESSMENTS

As training and recovery continue to progress, testing the body to ensure all is going well should remain an integral part of one's overall conditioning. It is also an important way to help maintain optimal training. The additional recommendations here are only a guide. It is always best to individualize them and with the help of a doctor or other healthcare professional. Some runners require different evaluations, while others will find these are adequate.

Daily Assessments

Morning Heart Rate. This is a general evaluation of one's autonomic nervous system—the important balance between the sympathetic and parasympathetic, and one of the ways the brain controls body function. As running progress is made, slow reductions in resting heart rate are expected, especially from improvements in cardiovascular health and increased circulation of blood through the aerobic muscles.

A simple way to monitor these changes is to check your morning heart rate. Strapping on a heart-rate monitor will give you an accurate reading. (The finger-on-the-wrist, or neck, to check for a pulse is not recommended for this evaluation.) Checking your morning heart rate before getting out of bed provides a true resting rate and good baseline, but checking it shortly upon getting up after sitting quietly for five minutes can serve the same purpose. Stick with the same routine each time.

The normal heart rate in the morning will vary. It should, however, be within the same range by about three to five beats on consecutive days. A change from one day to the next of more than about five or six beats per minute may be an indication that some type of stress is affecting the body. It may be an oncoming cold or flu, not enough sleep, early overtraining, or other issues. Perhaps your diet was not as good the previous day, or you've been allowing your heart rate to get too high on your aerobic workouts. It's a yellow cautionary flag and it should make you think about the cause of the elevated heart rate.

In a well-trained athlete, the pulse rate may be as low as the mid 30s, but many healthy athletes are in the 50s and 60s. What's more relevant is how it changes over time. As healthy training progresses, the pulse will gradually get lower. It's critical to note that lower is not necessarily better. In some individuals, a diminishing heart rate may indicate chronic overtraining.

Heart Rate Variability. In addition to resting heart rate, another important measurement is known as heart rate variability (HRV). It is the specific measurement of the time between each heartbeat. The heart normally speeds up when you inhale, and slows down on exhalation. A healthy, well-rested runner will produce a larger gap and higher HRV than someone with an overstressed body.

While a more detailed measurement of HRV is best achieved by a cardiologist using an ECG (electrocardiogram), today's technology allows anyone to measure HRV at home, using an iPhone or similar device. HRV is best evaluated in the morning when first waking up, although an evaluation performed after an aerobic run should demonstrate little or no stress. Yet following an anaerobic workout, the HRV usually indicates a certain degree of stress.

It is no surprise that runners who maintain a good balance of autonomic function, as indicated by HRV, perform better.

Body Weight. In a properly trained, healthy runner, there should be a slight loss of water weight during a long workout, such as a two-hour run. But if training stress elevates too much, and the brain's regulation of hormones impairs water and electrolyte balance, weight changes after a long run can become abnormal.

The pre- and post-weight evaluation should be made on a good quality scale following one's longest run of the week or month. Normally there may be up to a one to two percent drop in weight. More than this may indicate abnormal dehydration, which might be expected on dry sunny days with high heat. Otherwise it could indicate some metabolic imbalance.

A runner who gains weight during a long run is a sure sign of something wrong. In an unhealthy condition, the body holds more of the water consumed with long training. This is more commonly seen in a race, whereby athletes develop water intoxication associated with low blood sodium (hyponatremia). This problem is preventable, and only occurs in those who are unhealthy.

Blood, Urine and other Lab Tests

These evaluations vary with the individual. When all tests are normal, there is no need to perform them as often. However, when abnormal, re-evaluations more frequently would be important to assure whatever health improvements are being made are being realized. These are usually done in conjunction with a healthcare professional (although it is now possible for individuals to arrange for their own laboratory testing). Here are some of the common tests:

Blood. Various types of blood tests can be helpful and may include the following:

- A complete blood count (CBC) to monitor red cell count, hemoglobin, and hematocrit gives a more complete picture of physiological benefits. This also evaluates white blood cells.
- Testing key nutrients and related factors are important to do once or twice yearly, more if abnormalities are found. These include iron, ferritin, folic acid, vitamin B12, vitamin D, and other nutrients, along with sodium, magnesium and other electrolytes. Blood fats are important to measure too, including triglycerides, and the various types of cholesterol.
- The C-reactive protein (CRP) and erythrocyte sedimentation rate (ESR) are key tests to help rule out inflammation.
- Glycated hemoglobin (different from the CBC) can help determine the balance of blood sugar from previous months.
- Many other tests may be necessary as the individual's health dictates.

Urine. Testing the urine can also provide valuable information. Test strips available in drug and health stores may serve as a good general monthly test. These measure levels of protein, sugar, blood and other substances that may appear in urine. A health professional may also perform more extensive urine tests when needed, which can also provide information on hydration status.

Saliva. Scientists studying stress and the related hormone cortisol use saliva rather than blood to assess this substance. Salivary cortisol is performed four or more times over the course of a typical day and evening, rather than just once, for increased accuracy. In addition, blood tests for cortisol usually induce sufficient stress to temporarily raise this hormone, providing an inaccurate evaluation. Salivary tests are also available for other hormones too, including testosterone, the estrogens, and others.

The most important regular assessment that all runners should make on a regular basis is the maximum aerobic function (MAF) Test. It monitors the changes in training pace at the same sub-maximal heart rate. This is a measurement of what I call *aerobic speed*, and is the topic of the next chapter. Over the course of thirty-five years of coaching, I have used the MAF Test with thousands of runners, from world-champion endurance athletes such as six-time Hawaii Ironman champion Mark Allen to your typical recreational runner who wanted to lose weight, eliminate stress, improve performance, and run injury-free. I have also written extensively about the MAF Test in my earlier books and on my website.

The MAF Test is nothing new. That is, unless you have never tried it. Once you understand and apply the MAF Test to your own training and racing, you will wonder, "Why didn't I use this test before?" I imagine that almost all of the East African runners on the cusp of someday going 1:59 are unfamiliar with the MAF Test. But if they want to make marathon history by running several minutes faster, this simple test can help individualize their training.

CHAPTER 5

AEROBIC SPEED

Train, don't strain.

—ARTHUR LYDIARD, legendary New Zealand coach

The famously overused expression, "no pain, no gain," should have been retired long ago. These four words continue to have a toxic effect on most athletes, especially runners, whether competing on a world-class level or just hoping to finish their first marathon. No pain, no gain is so deeply engrained in almost every aspect of sports that a revolution in thinking is necessary for healthy, injury-free running. While I am just one voice, there are others who share my belief that *not* over-stressing the body is absolutely essential for safe conditioning and consistent racing.

It's important to train your body to run increasingly faster at a sub-maximal heart rate. The physiological reason is that 99 percent of the energy required for a marathon is generated by the body's aerobic system with one percent coming from its anaerobic counterpart. By building the body's diverse aerobic system for improved endurance and stamina, you can run at a faster pace—but smartly freed from pain. This will significantly improve running economy.

The sub-maximal level that I am using here varies with the individual. It is well below the VO_2max and lactate threshold, but slightly below the heart rate associated with one's marathon pace. It is about 80 to 85 percent of VO_2max. As I discuss later in this chapter, this level is the maximum aerobic heart rate and provides the best training stimulus to build a powerful aerobic system.

The body's aerobic system is not as well defined as the nervous system or intestines. Yet it's a significant component of many body functions ranging from heart and lungs to hormones and the brain. The aerobic system relies on the red muscle fibers (or cells), which make up the bulk of muscles for an endurance activity such as the marathon. These are sometimes referred to as *slow twitch* or just *aerobic* fibers. They support our joints and other physical structures, provide us with great endurance (versus sprint ability), and contain miles of important blood vessels. Most significantly, these fibers burn fat for fuel, and the reason they are called "fatigue-resistant." The aerobic muscles can help make the gait more efficient, prevent injuries, speed workout recovery, and keep the immune system, and the rest of the body, in a healthy state. Because improved aerobic function allows one to run faster at the same heart rate—reducing oxygen requirements—it can greatly increase running economy.

Don't be fooled by the word "slow" in slow twitch—these skeletal muscle fibers, which make up the bulk of those throughout the body, have the potential for great sub-max speed when they are well developed. A runner with a superb aerobic foundation will become physically and metabolically more efficient, much less prone to injury, stay healthy, and race faster. Developing the aerobic system to run faster at the same sub-max heart rate is referred to as *aerobic speed*.

Even before implementation of anaerobic training, or what is commonly known as speed work, and which I define as running above the sub-max level, a runner's increasing aerobic speed should also produce a faster race pace. It is even possible to predict performance from aerobic speed. Early in my career, I compared aerobic and race paces in hundreds of healthy runners over a period of several years. The results showed that more than 75 percent ran personal bests for a 5K or 10K on certified courses following a period of strict aerobic-only training that lasted between three and six months.

For a runner to break 14 minutes in the 5K, for example, one's aerobic pace would have to be about 5:30 minutes per mile, which would equate to a 4:30 race pace. Likewise, for a sub-30 minute 10K, an aerobic pace of around 5:15 would be necessary. This phenomenon also occurs for other endurance distances, including the marathon.

How fast will a runner's aerobic pace have to be to run a 1:59 marathon? While this can only be precisely answered after such a race, it can be estimated based on relationships between aerobic speed and race pace. One's marathon race pace appears to be about 15 to 20 seconds per mile faster than the maximum aerobic pace. Racing better than 4:35-mile pace 26.2 times is what's required for a 1:59 marathon. To accomplish this, an athlete would have to progress to about 4:50 to 4:55 minutes per mile at the maximum aerobic heart rate.

AEROBIC PACE AND PERFORMANCE

Here are several aerobic capacities and race results that I witnessed firsthand:

- In the early 1980s when I put a heart monitor on Norwegian Grete Waitz, who became a nine-time winner of the New York Marathon, she ran a 6:05 aerobic pace, which corresponded to her then 2:32 New York marathon—averaging 5:48 pace.
- Soon afterwards, I recorded a 5:00-mile aerobic pace for American Matt Centrowitz. This was good for a 13:12 5K, a national record.

- A few years later, England's Priscilla Welsh developed her aerobic pace to 6:00 minutes per mile, and ran a 2:30 marathon averaging 5:44 pace.
- Triathlete Mark Allen progressed to a 5:19 pace over a period of several years (beginning at an 8:20 pace at the same 155 heart rate). Although he ran a 29:59 10K on a certified road course, Mark's focus was the Hawaii Ironman Triathlon Championship, which he won six times. His sub-2:40 marathon (which included the bike-to-run transition time) in 1996 is a record that still stands today.

Developing top aerobic speed begins with determining the proper training heart rate. Choosing a rate that is too high, even by a couple of beats, can increase the production of the stress hormone cortisol in a runner's body. Cortisol is produced by the adrenal glands under the direction of the brain when the amount of strain on the body is too high. This stress hormone can impair aerobic function, and cause a number of other problems including muscle imbalance, reduced fat burning, and irregularities in other hormones such as testosterone.

Choosing a training heart rate that is too low does not allow for maximum development of aerobic speed.

MAXIMUM AEROBIC HEART RATE

Since 1977, I have been assessing, treating, and coaching athletes on all levels. This involved employing a wide variety of assessment procedures to help find a particular level of training intensity that would produce optimal gains in the aerobic system while minimizing the stresses that could impair it. When successful, it is evidenced by significant improvements in aerobic speed, reductions in RQ indicating increased fat burning, balanced hormone levels, optimization of gait, and better race performance. This level of training is associated with the maximum aerobic heart rate.

When I was working with athletes, determining the maximum aerobic HR was highly individualized. It began with an extensive assessment process that included a detailed history of fitness (training and racing patterns), health (any illnesses), stress factors, and a complete inventory of signs and symptoms of injuries. This was followed by a physical evaluation, which provided information on muscle balance, bone health, foot function, and other aspects of biomechanics. There was also an evaluation of posture and gait, and it entailed treadmill and track assessment at the full spectrum of one's heart rate. Blood and urine tests were commonly employed, as was an extensive dietary analysis.

Long before there were wireless heart rate monitors, I relied on a bulky device used in hospitals for cardiac patients. There were wide elastic bands that strapped around the chest and shoulder, but it was effective in displaying an accurate heart rate for use on the treadmill, track and roads.

In some runners, it took a few days or weeks at this training level to determine that a slow, gradual accumulation of stress had occurred, and this meant a need to reduce the previously determined max aerobic heart rate.

In addition, one's pace should gradually improve as indicated by running faster at the same maximum aerobic HR. In particular, the pace should not slow down. This became one of the most important assessment tools.

The process of determining an athlete's maximum aerobic HR was tedious because of the one-on-one time involved, although rewarding. It is typical for the practice of individualization. Wanting to share these procedures with others who could not obtain such an evaluation, I separately developed the "180 formula." By considering a variety of factors, from age to injury history, an athlete could determine his or her own individual maximum aerobic heart rate that would be very close or identical to what I would find through extensive evaluations.

The 220 Heart Rate Formula had been commonly used for years, and I initially used it as a guideline. However, the training HR I found to be ideal in my assessment was often very different from the 220 Formula—usually significantly lower. In addition, it was becoming evident that athletes who regularly used the 220 Formula heart rate during training showed poor gait, increased muscle imbalance, and other problems following a workout at that heart rate, and that these athletes were more often injured or overtrained.

THE 180 FORMULA

To find your max aerobic HR, there are two important steps. First, subtract your age from 180. Next, find the best category for your present state of fitness and health, and make the appropriate adjustments:

1. Subtract your age from 180.
2. Modify this number by selecting among the following categories the one that best matches your fitness and health profile:
   a) If you have or are recovering from a major illness (heart disease, any operation or hospital stay, etc.) or are on any regular medication, subtract an additional 10.

b) If you are injured, have regressed in training or competition, get more than two colds or bouts of flu per year, have allergies or asthma, or if you have been inconsistent or are just getting back into training, subtract an additional 5.

c) If you have been training consistently (at least four times weekly) for up to two years without any of the problems just mentioned, keep the number (180–age) the same.

d) If you have been training for more than two years without any of the problems listed above, and have made progress in competition without injury, add 5.

For example, if you are thirty years old and fit into category (b), you get the following:

180–30=150. Then 150–5=145 beats per minute (bpm).

In this example, 145 will be the highest heart rate for all training, allowing you to most efficiently build an aerobic base. Training above this heart rate rapidly incorporates anaerobic function, exemplified by a shift to burning more sugar and less fat for fuel.

If it is difficult to decide which of two groups best fits you, then choose the group or outcome that results in the lower heart rate. For runners who have special circumstances not discussed here, further individualization with the help of a healthcare practitioner or other specialist familiar with your circumstance and knowledgeable in endurance sports may be necessary.

Two situations may be exceptions to the above calculations:

- The 180 Formula may need to be further individualized for people over the age of sixty-five. For some of these athletes, up to 10 beats may have to be added for those in category (d) in the 180 Formula, and depending on individual levels of fitness and health. This does not mean 10 should automatically be added, but that an honest self-assessment is important.

- For runners sixteen years of age and under, the formula is not applicable; rather, a heart rate of 165 may be best.

Once a maximum aerobic HR is found, a range from this heart rate to 10 beats below could be used for training. For example, if a runner's heart rate is determined to be 155, the aerobic training zone would be 145 to 155 beats per minute. However, the more training at 155, the quicker the aerobic system will be developed.

As you can see, the 180 Formula does not consider resting or maximum heart rates because it factors in other, more important health and fitness variables.

MAXIMUM AEROBIC FUNCTION (MAF) TEST

It is important to objectively assess the progress of the aerobic system, or more specifically that of aerobic speed. Using basic biofeedback, it is possible to measure changes in pace at a consistent heart rate on a track or road. This evaluates a runner's maximum aerobic function.

As the months pass, a runner can continually train faster at sub-maximal efforts, and stay healthy and injury-free. This involves testing a runner's *maximum aerobic function*, called MAF. It is usually performed on a track, where five, one-mile splits at the maximum aerobic HR are recorded.

I recommended performing this test monthly, although when training on the same road course, it is easy for a runner to evaluate the pace each day, making sure it was at least as fast as previous runs.

Here is the MAF Test protocol:

- The Test begins with an easy warm up at a lower intensity. One's heart rate should slowly be raised during gradual increases in speed. The maximum aerobic HR is reached only after 15 minutes or more. The warm-up prepares the body for the main part of the workout. It increases blood flow into the aerobic muscles, raises blood fats for use as fuel, improves lung capacity, increases flexibility, and other important benefits.
- The warm-up is followed by the main part of the MAF Test. This involves running continuously for five miles on the track, while maintaining the max aerobic HR. Each mile split is recorded.
- Test results should be carefully recorded each month.

Below are the results of a 30-year-old male runner's first MAF Test 1, and the results of another recorded four months later (Test 5). The test was performed while maintaining a heart rate of 148 (and all training between the two tests was at or below 148).

MAF Test 1

Mile 1	6:07
Mile 2	6:11
Mile 3	6:18
Mile 4	6:26
Mile 5	6:37

MAF Test 5

Mile 1	5:34
Mile 2	5:34
Mile 3	5:37
Mile 4	5:39
Mile 5	5:41

As the weeks pass, the MAF Test should demonstrate increases in pace. In addition, differences between the first and fifth mile should be less. Both occurred in the MAF Test on the above runner.

While a monthly assessment such as this one is important, observing improvement can often be seen during regular workouts. During a run on a familiar course, for example, the same type of general assessment can be made. One-mile splits are not necessarily required. A ten-mile loop, for example, that is run at one's max aerobic HR, will take less time to complete with each passing week, factoring in the warm up (and cool down). So almost every day, the runner will have a good sense of whether the body is training at least as well or better than yesterday or last week. However, I still recommend performing an MAF Test on the track every month, which provides a consistent, more controlled assessment on the same flat accurate course.

During the MAF Test, it is important to choose days with similar conditions. Temperature, humidity, precipitation, and wind can all affect the aerobic pace. Extremes of certain conditions, such as high heat and humidity verses cooler, dry days, could affect the MAF Test outcomes by 10, 15, or more seconds per mile. In addition, wearing the same lightweight shoes, such as racing flats, for each test is recommended as other overly supported, cushioned shoes could result in a slightly slower pace. When recording MAF Tests, it is critical to note any significant weather differences, shoes or other factors that may vary from one test to another, including how you feel.

MAF REGRESSION

As with any assessment, there may be indications that progress has stalled, or even that the aerobic pace is slowing. Regression of the aerobic pace is usually a significant indication of something going wrong in the physical, chemical or mental aspects of the body. Observing a higher than normal morning heart rate can be an early warning sign.

If the aerobic pace slows, or, as in some cases, fails to improve, it is prudent to immediately reduce training until the underlying cause, or causes, are found. In this situation, decreasing training by 30 to 50 percent is highly advised. Outside assistance from a coach or healthcare professional may be very helpful in determining what factors are impairing the aerobic system. The chart below lists some common problems.

SOME FACTORS THAT IMPAIR AEROBIC PROGRESS

1. Training with too high a maximum aerobic HR. This happens if the initial assessment was improperly performed.
2. Allowing the training HR to rise above the maximum aerobic level during training. This may occur when ascending a steep hill without reducing the pace, or training with others who are running faster. For some runners, even slight elevations in heart rate can add stress to the body, most especially when health is not optimal.
3. Infections, including bacterial and viral. Sometimes the only evidence of this is an elevated temperature, even slightly.
4. Nutritional imbalance. Poor iron status, for example, reduces the function of the red aerobic muscle fibers. A pre-workout meal high in carbohydrates, which elevates insulin and reduces fat burning, can diminish aerobic function and pace.

5. The accumulation of physical, chemical and mental stress can elevate the hormone cortisol, reducing fat burning and aerobic function.
6. Muscle imbalance can reduce the economy of one's gait, raising the heart rate and forcing the pace to decrease.
7. Anaerobic training can impair the aerobic system. This can include racing, interval workouts, weight lifting or combinations of these. During the period of building the aerobic system, it is vital to avoid these types of workouts until an effective aerobic system is developed.

It is important to allow the aerobic system sufficient time to build a solid foundation. This period of training has been called an *aerobic base*, where all workouts should be run at the max aerobic HR.

When one first starts running at the maximum aerobic HR, the common reaction is often, "Hey, I can't believe I'm running so slowly. I better speed up!" Runners feel the pace is subjectively slow, because they often train above this HR, and having to back off from their usual pace makes them feel the workout is somehow less effective. Peer pressure often plays a role. It is sometimes best to train alone during this period. Being patient will reap great aerobic benefits.

But as the aerobic system continues developing, speed increases at the same heart rate. Over time, the pace quickens, and many runners now feel it is a bit challenging because of the fast pace—despite being at the same heart rate. This is particularly true for runs over ninety minutes in duration. This level of progress, which should begin early in the program, may take several weeks or months depending on the athlete.

If the MAF Tests show an increase in aerobic speed each month, you should still continue with only aerobic training, and not exceed the maximum aerobic HR during any workouts. As this aerobic pace quickens, so does race pace.

As daily workouts become faster and more physically demanding, maintaining these paces for extended periods of time during each workout may be difficult. This is the time for alternating hard-easy days, or using *fartlek* workouts (running by feel)—but always at or below the max aerobic HR. An option I have found to be very successful is to perform *aerobic intervals,* where one runs a slower pace for a few minutes, then runs at the max aerobic pace for a few minutes, then recovers again with a slower pace. Here's an example of such a workout:

- Warm up 15 or more minutes.
- Run at the max aerobic HR; in this example, the runner can maintain 5:30 pace with relative comfort for about 20 minutes.
- Reduce the pace to 6:15, or some relatively easy recovery pace, for about 10 minutes, more if needed.
- Return to the max aerobic HR for another 20 minutes.
- Continue alternating an easier pace with the max aerobic level for the duration of the workout.
- Cool down for at least 15 minutes.

There's another workout that allows runners to reach their race pace without the HR exceeding the max aerobic level. This is the downhill MAF run. Find a course with a long downhill grade, ranging from 200 meters to a mile or more. The grade should not be so steep as to disturb one's gait, but steep enough to allow for a faster pace at the same max aerobic HR. (A course with a shorter downhill section can be turned into one of the downhill MAF repeats.) This workout might look like this:

- Warm up for at least 15 minutes.
- Run the downhill section at the max aerobic HR. Due to gravity, this results in a faster-than-normal pace. The perfect grade is one that results in running at or just above race pace. But it is essential to maintain a good gait—avoid over-striding or heel striking.
- Remain on the hilly course or perform downhill repeats as the terrain dictates.
- Cool down for at least 15 minutes.

By building a strong and fast aerobic system, fat burning increases, physical injuries can be prevented, and running economy—often the missing link in enhancing performance—can improve significantly.

MAF Test vs. Running Race Pace

The chart shows some compilations for 5K races.

MAF Pace	5K Race Pace	5K Time
10:00	7:30	23:18
9:00	7:00	21:45
8:30	6:45	20:58
8:00	6:30	20:12
7:30	6:00	18:38
7:00	5:30	17:05
6:30	5:15	16:19
6:00	5:00	15:32
5:45	4:45	14:45
5:30	4:30	13:59
5:15	4:20	13:28
5:00	4:15	13:12

ANAEROBIC TRAINING

Some runners are blessed with natural true speed—sprinters and to a large degree those with great 5K and 10K times. At least, they will be faster in relation to their peers as they age. If one builds health and remains fit, this type of power remains, and the brain always knows how to run relatively fast. This means a 13-minute 5K runner will remain fast years later, relative to those that he raced against when younger. Of course, this runner won't run at the same pace as in his prime.

The thirty-five-year old runner who used to clock fast 5K or 10K times at his peak may never become as fast at these distances. Rather, longer distances will be where improvement can best be achieved, because building a strong aerobic foundation is more about training and less about genetic inheritance. This helps explain why many elite marathoners in their late 20s and early 30s, who were once equally fast middle-distance runners, may turn out to be the best candidates for a 1:59 marathon.

Building a strong aerobic base with its accompanying aerobic speed can help anyone run a faster marathon because of improved running economy. In particular, it can provide the necessary edge for elite marathoners, who are already running under 2:06, to shave several minutes off their times.

That is not to say I don't recommend anaerobic training, whether interval workouts, weights, or other approaches to building the anaerobic system. However, the addition of harder training can potentially cause a plateau or regression of aerobic speed. This problem can occur with too much anaerobic work, and is usually visible by monitoring daily runs, and quite clear from the MAF Test. The reason for this stagnation or downturn is partly related to the stress response by the body following anaerobic efforts. The frequently increased production of the stress hormone cortisol can impair fat burning and aerobic function. (The measurement of salivary cortisol is an effective way to assess overall stress.)

Anaerobic training also increases oxidative stress—the production of dangerous chemicals throughout the body. This can impair aerobic function by adversely affecting the mitochondria—the powerhouse of the red, aerobic muscle fiber, where fat is converted to energy. Oxidative stress is also associated with overtraining.

If stress begins to affect the aerobic system, the runner may initially feel fine. But if the stress is allowed to continue, then this can lead to poor performance, injury, or poor health.

Many runners believe the addition of anaerobic training will help them perform better in a marathon. This may or may not be true, depending on the individual. I have seen many great marathon performances from those who only have trained at their maximum aerobic paces.

One option for runners who want to add anaerobic work into their schedules is to race shorter distances. Depending on the individual, a 10K, 15K, or half-marathon provide at least two important benefits. First, these races can be a good anaerobic workout. As such, it can encourage the development of the anaerobic system, as little as is necessary for running a great marathon. A second benefit might include racing at the end of one's aerobic-only base period. It can be an eye-opener, helping to break the long-standing traditional notion that to race fast one must train fast with anaerobic intervals.

Accomplishing a 1:59 marathon will require a runner to have outstanding aerobic speed, along with other critical factors that improve running economy. As long as our elite runner avoids the trap of

How Old Will the First 1:59 Marathoner Be?

I will continue mentioning thirty-something-year-old runners in the same context of a 1:59 marathoner. It is possible that the optimal age group for this feat will be runners between thirty and thirty-seven, possibly even older. This is when the body's endurance capabilities potentially have matured: aerobic pace has grown faster, fat burning is better, more efficient gait has evolved, and, just as importantly, there is more marathon experience. Over the past two decades, the average age of the top international marathoners is around thirty years. The very best ones may be slightly older. Ethiopia's Haile Gebrselassie was thirty-five when he set a world record in 2008. (After that race, he told the press he was too old to run a 1:59 marathon.) Portugal's Carlos Lopes was thirty-seven when he won the marathon at the 1984 Los Angeles Olympics. The following year, Lopes triumphed at the Rotterdam Marathon, setting a new world record of 2:07:12, nearly a minute faster than the current fastest time. Then there's Meb. Keflezighi was one month shy of turning thirty-nine when he won the 2014 Boston Marathon.

The risk for veteran or "older" marathoners is the common problem of chronic injuries. This can be a result of overtraining because many runners and coaches think training should proceed at the same level as it did years earlier. A lot more rest and recovery is necessary.

overtraining, the odds of making marathon history increases. So let's look more closely at what is meant by overtraining—the subject of the next chapter.

Chapter 6

Overreaching vs. Overtraining

The secret is simple, train, train and train more.
> —Geoffrey Mutai, a Kenyan, with fastest marathon
> time ever, at 2011 Boston Marathon, and 2013
> New York City Marathon winner

Why are America's top professional marathoners frequently getting injured? It's a fair question to ask, since many of us are waiting for the next Frank Shorter to take gold in the Olympic marathon or a Bill Rodgers to dominate Boston or New York City. Ryan Hall and Dathan Ritzenhein were slated to become America's best hope of taking on the East Africans, of giving them a real taste of competition. While both runners have churned out many great races—and victories—at various distances, neither has shown long-term consistency due to lingering injuries and illnesses.

In the 2008 Beijing Olympic Marathon, Ritzenhein was the top US runner, finishing ninth with a time of 2:11:59. At the 2012 Chicago Marathon, where he set a new personal record of 2:07:47, he again placed ninth and was the fastest non-African runner. But over the years, the former American record-holder in the 5,000 meters (12:56.27) has dealt with a bout of pneumonia, a stress fracture in his foot, and then a nasty foot wound that kept him sidelined from training and competition for six months.

In the 2012 Olympic Marathon Trials, Ritzenhein placed a disappointing fourth and failed to make the marathon squad, though he finished thirteenth in the 10,000 meters Olympic finals with a time of 27:45.89 behind winner Mo Farah (27:30:42) and second-place US finisher Galen Rupp (27:30:90), who is now one of the country's leading distance specialists. (In January 2014, Rupp set the American record in the Indoor 2-Mile with a time of 8:07.41.)

In a 2012 interview with *Running Times*, Ritzehheim, who was being coached by Alberto Salazar, admitted that "there's no lie; I've had a lot of injuries. My body felt banged up. I was always dancing around little problems, and I'm trying to be a lot more proactive on it now. We were always trying to chase a reason for an injury, and we did find some problems, but there were other problems that we were looking at—real obvious things—instead of built-up injury patterns."

Ryan Hall, who holds the US record in the half-marathon (59:43), was the first American runner to crack the one-hour barrier in the event. At the 2011 Boston Marathon, Hall ran the fastest marathon ever by an American, 2:04:58, to finish fourth. But since that jaw-dropping performance, his career has been plagued by injuries. One of the pre-race favorites for a medal at the London Olympic Marathon, he pulled up lame at the eleven-mile mark with a hamstring injury. In 2013, Hall was slated to run the Boston Marathon and New York City Marathons, but withdrew from both races due to another injury. In a press release announcing his withdrawal from New York, the two-time Olympian said the following:

In my zealous efforts to have redemption in this year's ING New York City Marathon, I overstepped the first and most important rule—making it to the line healthy. A long string of very aggressive training has aggravated my hip and it has not been able to fully calm down, such that I don't think racing on it is wise. I am very disappointed that I won't be lining up on November 3rd as I had so looked forward to, but I am refocusing now on getting back to 100 percent.

Determined to reclaim his marathon mojo, Hall, now 31, proceeded to scale back his high-mileage training by substituting quality over quantity. But after a promising start at the 2014 Boston Marathon, he faded badly and ran a very disappointing 2:17:50, finishing twentieth overall and behind *nine* other American runners. Did his career peak several years ago?

No one likes to see talented runners prematurely realize that perhaps their best racing days might be in the past. But are elite runners more susceptible to injuries? What is the long-term, cumulative effect of "aggressive training?"

Based on my own personal experience, I believe that it is entirely possible for the very best runners to stay healthy and injury-free, and even get faster deep into their late thirties. Almost all of the problems that great runners develop over time, including but not limited to stress fractures, hamstring or back issues, and lingering respiratory ailments, are completely preventable. Running is not a contact sport like football, so when problems arise, it is an indication that something has gone wrong in training, diet, or lifestyle. The remedy is to locate the underlying cause of the problem, fix it, and then resume optimal training and racing.

For elite runners who depend on sponsorships, appearance fees, and prize money to sustain their livelihood, the demands of their sport require the artful balancing of knowing when to push hard *and* when to ease off in training. Each runner must find that sweet spot, either alone or in consultation with one's coach, trainer, or therapist. Locating that sweet spot isn't always immediately apparent; it's hidden within a gray area between overreaching and overtraining.

One of the greatest impediments to a 1:59 marathon will be overtraining. On the other hand, accomplishing it can be achieved through overreaching—OR—which is defined here as the highest level of training, in volume and/or intensity, that one can reach and still be able to progress and properly recover. Without experiencing OR, a runner most likely will never achieve true athletic potential. But the real challenge exists on the opposite end of the training spectrum—overtraining, or OT. This is where too many runners cross that Rubicon line from OR. They overshoot the body's limits and fall by the side of the road, beaten, worn down, injured, and doubtful about their future in the sport.

The full spectrum of training

undertraining   overreaching   overtraining
                        "sweet spot"

There are many markers and symptoms of overtraining, but these unfortunately can be elusive at the onset. Only when one feels completely boxed in or affected by these symptoms, do the signs of OT become most apparent. Injury, mood changes, poor sleep, and various health issues, ranging from infections to asthma and allergies to chronic inflammation in joints, muscles or even body-wide fatigue, not to mention poor performances, only begin to describe OT's consequences. The chart here lists some of these common complaints.

POSSIBLE SIGNS AND SYMPTOMS ASSOCIATED WITH OVERTRAINING

Signs:
Hormone imbalance
Chronic inflammation
Low blood sodium
Increased infections
Poor sleep
Elevated blood lactate
Reduced heart rate variability
Blood-sugar irregularity
Poor Maximum Aerobic Function (MAF) Tests
Reduced or plateau in performance

Symptoms:
Mental or physical fatigue
Pain in muscles and joints
Physical injury
Asthma or allergy
Mood changes
Anxiety
Feeling of overall body weakness

An ongoing elevated resting heart rate is a red-flag warning that a runner has entered the early stages of OT. The Maximum Aerobic Function (MAF) Test is an effective indicator of OT (see previous chapter), because training heart rates also rise. Those runners who regularly monitor their aerobic-training workouts would usually observe a slowing of pace at the same heart rate as the first indication of possible OT.

There are other clues as to whether a runner is overtraining. In 2012, Yann Le Meur and colleagues at the National Institute of the Sport in Paris, France, published their study on overtraining in endurance athletes using a multidisciplinary approach. Of the many signs and symptoms (similar to those noted here), elevations in lactate and heart rate were most effective in determining OT.

Due to an incomplete understanding of the relationship between OR and OT, runners often seek treatment for an injury after the fact. By then, it might be too late because the damage has already been done. But one simple fact is clear: the causes of OT almost always include too much running and too little recovery.

To remain healthy and injury-free, follow this simple equation: Training = Workout + Rest

Increased training is best tolerated through interspersed periods of recovery that are sometimes referred to as periodization. Careful training, including longer runs, builds the body's aerobic system and contributes to the ability to race faster. However, that's only half the formula for optimal performance.

Just as important as training is recovery. It is easy to push through the workouts, especially when running with others, watched by a coach or following a program with specific time or mileage goals to meet. But due to outside pressure, usually a result of comparing one's training with others, or maybe it's a reaction to internal psychological demands, rest and recovery seem to be taken less seriously. Taking time off, even for a day or two, is also considered a weakness, a flaw in the runner's character.

This mindset usually starts early on if one shows promise as a runner; it may be reinforced by high school and college track coaches who are the so-called high priests of "no pain, no gain." Yet it doesn't have to be that way. "No one will burn out doing aerobic running," said Arthur Lydiard. "It is too much anaerobic running, which the American scholastic athletic system tends to put young athletes through that burns them out."

What is overlooked is that most training benefits actually take place during the period of recovery. With the right training, rest allows the body to improve.

Let's take a closer look at the training formula:

$$Training = Workout + Rest$$

Altering the training equation often leads to either undertraining or overtraining. For those seeking peak performance, making sure this equation is balanced is essential—it's a significant factor for anyone seeking a 1:59 marathon, or a PR in any race. An imbalance in the training equation produces physical, chemical and mental-emotional stress. In fact, the issue of overtraining is one of excess stress beyond which the body is less able to cope. Lifestyle factors, especially stress, also influence OT. The sidebar below discusses the critical features of excess stress.

PHYSICAL, CHEMICAL, AND MENTAL STRESS

Our scientific knowledge about stress began in the 1920s, when famous stress-research pioneer Hans Selye began to piece together the common problems resulting from excessive stress. These include the adrenal gland, immune and intestinal dysfunction, which in turn can trigger a variety of symptoms. Stress can quickly impair running performance, and follow the same stages as overtraining.

There are three types of stress that can contribute to OT.

Physical Stress

Physical stresses are strains or exertions on the body that many runners take for granted. Disturbing the delicate training equation—too much training and/or too little rest—can quickly introduce physical stress on muscles, joints, bones and other body parts. Other significant physical stresses can include wearing shoes that don't fit just right, too much sitting, dental problems, and muscle imbalance.

Chemical Stress

Many chemicals from our environment can adversely affect the body, causing stress. These include air and water pollution, preservatives and additives in foods, household chemicals and toiletries such as cleaning products, soaps, and cosmetics, and many others. Low levels of vitamin D (not enough sunlight) is a common example of a chemical stress. In addition, drugs can induce stress. Included are excess caffeine or alcohol, or the side effects of prescription or over-the-counter drugs such as painkillers. These chemicals can influence your heart rate, breathing, immune system, intestines, muscles, and function of the brain. Reducing harmful chemicals from air, water, and food, and improving diet quality are key ways to reducing this form of stress. Chemical stresses can also affect physical and mental-emotional problems.

Mental and Emotional Stress

The mental and emotional state includes the behavioral aspects of our brains. The mental condition may be referred to as cognition, which involves sensation, perception, learning, concept formation, and decision-making. Overtraining can impair this component of the brain. The emotional state typically describes pain, moods of anxiety or depression, and loss of enthusiasm or motivation—symptoms common in overtrained runners.

A multitude of physical, chemical and mental/emotional stress can come from various sources—career, family, other people, infections, allergic reactions, and even the weather. Most runners are affected by more than one form of stress, and frequently by all three types. Stress is also cumulative. The response to a physical stress from the weekend's 10K race can become magnified by Monday's chemically-related stress of too much coffee and poor eating, further compounded by pressure from work or family-related emotional stress later in the week. All of this may affect one's brain and body by the following weekend with symptoms of fatigue, headache, or intestinal distress.

What's important to realize about stress is that too much of it interferes with rest. Or more accurately, recovering from excess stress requires additional down time. If you don't get enough rest, usually in the form of sleep, the effects of stress will continue to accumulate. Unfortunately, one problem associated with stress is that it can contribute to insomnia, maintaining a vicious stress cycle.

Quality sleep is a powerful stress remedy. This means a minimum of about eight hours of uninterrupted sleep each night. But as training volume and/or intensity rises to higher levels, this amount of sleep may not be enough—another hour or two, which may include a daily nap, may be necessary. Those who still require more sleep may be in the early stage of OT.

Like most physiological processes, training is located on a single spectrum as shown on page 78. At one end is a deficiency, typically seen in underactive people with low fitness and motivation. It also applies to casual athletes who are unable or unwilling to train sufficient hours to perform to their potential. The opposite end of the spectrum is overtraining. A third to half of runners may fall into this state at various times during their highly competitive years, with some studies claiming the figure at 60 percent.

While the most common cause of OT is usually an imbalance of training and recovery, various lifestyle factors may also exist. These include dietary problems that can adversely affect running, such as insufficient nutritional intake, including total calories, and foods containing healthy fat and quality protein. Job stress can be another significant contributor to OT. For pro runners, this may include dealing with the non-running business side of the sport—finding or holding onto sponsorships, frequent travel, and appearances at marathon expos.

With too much running, or insufficient recovery or some combination of the two, possibly in conjunction with other stresses, two important and interrelated aspects of the body are adversely affected leading to OT:

- The brain
- The hormones

When confronted by OT, the body relies on an important mechanism that incorporates these two aspects in its attempt to adapt to this stress. It is called the hypothalamic-pituitary-adrenal axis.

THE HYPOTHALAMIC-PITUITARY-ADRENAL AXIS

The brain plays a major role in regulating stress throughout the body. This is also an essential way to recover from training and racing. The brain influences muscle function, energy production, water regulation, electrolyte balance, as well as the glands that produce the hormones. This process of adapting begins in a small region of the brain called the hypothalamus. With its information about the status of the body, the brain directs the pituitary gland, housed in the middle of the organ, to produce a variety of hormones that are sent to the body for repair and rebuilding. The pituitary is also influenced by memories and emotions stored in nearby regions of the brain.

The pituitary releases hormones that stimulate the body's other glands, in particular those of the adrenals, to control metabolism, muscle function, and sex hormones, including testosterone, vital for healthy muscles. Often referred to as the "master gland," the pituitary has significant control over one's entire hormonal system, and helps funnel information to it from the brain.

The pituitary also secretes growth hormone, which stimulates muscle development. Its production occurs during sleep. While the amount of growth hormone made is higher in childhood and is reduced as one ages, sufficient amounts are still secreted even in older, healthy individuals. Like other hormones naturally produced in the body, poor health and inadequate sleep may reduce the level of growth hormone.

Unfortunately, it's become too common for those seeking to restore youth, control weight, or enhance sports performance to also take human growth hormone (HGH). However, the use of HGH does not actually guarantee more muscles or improved performance. It's a banned substance in sports, and its use is dangerous. Taking it can reduce the pituitary's ability to produce growth hormone, creating an even more serious problem when HGH ingestion is stopped. Taking HGH can also cause side effects that include fatigue, muscle weakness, reduced sex hormones and sexual function, and blood-sugar irregularities.

By avoiding the pitfalls of OT, runners can progress unimpeded and more easily reach their athletic potential. Unfortunately, too many fall into the OT trap.

Through my own research, I have delineated three stages of what is best referred to as the *overtraining syndrome*. (A syndrome is a set of signs and symptoms associated with some disorder. It is usually individual: some runners have certain OT indications and not others, with the opposite true in other athletes.)

As OT develops, the brain may be unable to maintain proper body balance. This results in specific signs and symptoms throughout the body, which can be broken into three stages.

STAGE 1 OVERTRAINING

This first stage of OT is associated with an excess stimulation of the sympathetic nervous system. Imagine having a couple of large espressos before your run (perhaps you already do this). It makes you feel good and helps you run better, so you think. But your heart rate rises due to the stress of caffeine. This is a high sympathetic state, which can temporarily improve strength. Some runners are already in this state—this stimulation is ongoing. Even upon waking, resting heart rate is higher than usual.

For some runners, one result of this early sympathetic over-activity is a sudden, short-lived improvement in performance—significant enough to have a breakthrough race or two. This usually encourages more of the same training, mistakenly believing one is on the right path. But if OT is not quickly reversed, performance turns poor.

I am sometimes asked if a runner can be "overtrained" into a strong, record-setting performance. But the more important question is: Should a runner put his health in jeopardy for the sake of being the first to go 1:59? I would never participate in such an activity or endeavor—it is unwise, grossly unethical, and could cause significant harm to the runner. My steadfast rule in coaching has always been to never sacrifice an athlete's health for increased fitness and speed. One can equally have great races with proper training, improved health, careful assessments, and patience.

The onset of Stage 1 OT may not be accompanied by obvious signs or symptoms, at least initially, but rather, by very subtle or sub-clinical ones. The most common is an abnormal plateau or regression in the MAF Test, indicating the start of reduced aerobic function and fat burning (also observed as an elevated RQ at specific sub-max heart rates). In addition, the resting heart rate may begin to elevate.

In many cases, other evaluations, such as blood or urine tests, appear normal.

But if Stage 1 continues to progress, running economy quickly diminishes. This is most evident by the presence of more noticeable reductions in pace at the same sub-max heart rate. It is also associated with irregularities in the running gait, and even resting posture.

Physical and mental fatigue, cognitive impairment, physical injury, sleeping irregularities, abnormal hunger, or cravings, especially for sweets and refined carbohydrates, and other complaints may develop as a result.

In addition, in an attempt to respond to OT, an elevation of the stress hormone cortisol is produced by the adrenal glands. This is the result of messages from the brain (via the pituitary), a call for more help in adapting the body to the stress of OT. High cortisol puts the body into a high-alert stress state, and can reduce fat burning and impair aerobic function, along with other problems that can compromise the immune system and the intestines.

With both an overactive sympathetic nervous system, and high levels of cortisol, other problems can develop. These might include:

- Muscle imbalance (detailed in Chapter 8) causing reduced joint flexibility, pain or other common injuries especially in the back, knees, ankles, and feet.
- Storage of more body fat and possible weight gain.
- Other hormone-related problems can arise in both men and women.
- Reduced sexual desire, with infertility in some cases.
- Mental and emotional stress such as depression and anxiety.

Overtraining must be corrected by addressing its cause, whether too much training volume or intensity, too little rest, other lifestyle factors, or, as is often the case, some combination of problems. Otherwise, the situation worsens and the athlete can enter stage two.

STAGE 2 OVERTRAINING

Many healthcare professionals, coaches, trainers, and athletes recognize the second stage of OT because the condition is now more obvious. Specifically, the overactive sympathetic system and high cortisol continue to adversely affect the body and brain, especially impairing the aerobic system. The significant elevation in the resting and training heart rate further worsens the MAF Test.

Stage 2 OT is more common in runners with a moderate to high level of anaerobic training as a significant part of their workout schedules. This may include interval workouts on the track, too much racing, and improper weight training.

High cortisol further disturbs the balance of other hormones. For example, it can increase insulin levels, reducing fat burning with increased fat storage. It can lower testosterone and DHEA, both important for muscle recovery. Other hormone imbalance can also result in the excess loss of sodium from the body. Too low a level of sodium in the blood, which is also called hyponatremia, may be associated with water intoxication. This goes beyond poor racing; it is a serious health problem that could even cause death.

Fortunately, this particular stage on the OT spectrum can be corrected. It will take longer to recover, but all aspects of excess stress must be assessed and remedied. This includes restricting training to only aerobic workouts, avoiding all anaerobic efforts, including racing, and making other important changes with diet and lifestyle as needed.

Those who don't listen to their body and continue OT can have worsening signs and symptoms, including reduction in performance and development of more debilitating chronic injuries. Many runners remain stuck in this stage of overtraining for months and even years. Worse, some progress into the more serious third stage of OT.

STAGE 3 OVERTRAINING

Chronic OT can lead to more serious brain, muscle, and metabolic problems. These signs and symptoms continue to parallel chronic adrenal and other hormone imbalances, further reduction in the aerobic system, and a disturbed hypothalamic-pituitary-adrenal axis. Eventually, the body becomes so exhausted, that many hormones can no longer maintain normal levels.

In the adrenal glands, for example, the ability to produce cortisol is nearly lost. The result is just the opposite from Stages 1 and 2— abnormally low cortisol. This contributes to a worsening physical, chemical, and mental condition.

The once overactive sympathetic system has become exhausted, and now there is an abnormally low resting heart rate. This is the result of the parasympathetic nervous system dominating. Just getting out of bed in the morning becomes difficult. However, the MAF

Test has usually regressed dramatically as the training heart rate is high.

Stage 3 is typically accompanied by the lack of desire to compete and sometimes train and race. Depression, significant injury, and most notably severe exhaustion are common. Performance may diminish considerably and many runners in this state consider themselves sidelined, burned out, or may even quietly retire from competitive sports.

The chronic hormonal problems can continue to increase sodium loss, further raising the runner's vulnerability to hyponatremia, water intoxication, and brain injury.

Athletes who are in the third stage of overtraining are seriously unwell, and should seek help from a healthcare professional. Many are at high risk for chronic diseases of the heart, blood vessels, pancreas, and other areas. Recovery and return to previous optimal levels of performance is a very difficult task.

Overtraining is preventable. Through effective, ongoing assessments, especially the MAF Test, runners can monitor themselves to progress into overreaching and avoid entering OT. Instead, by remaining in the OR state, there are a number of elite, world-class runners who have the potential to run 1:59.

CHAPTER 7

TRAINING SCHEDULES

I think the job toughened me up, climbing and walking and stooping all day. When I began my run at night, I was tired; but after a mile or so, the tiredness went away.

—JOHNNY KELLEY, two-time Boston Marathon winner (1935, 1945), who also competed in the race sixty-one times, commenting on his job as a maintenance worker at Boston Edison Electric Company

Far too many runners are obsessed with following strict training schedules. Any small deviation from planned workouts fills them with anxiety. There's the usual concern that not meeting weekly mileage totals can lead to poor racing. Running magazines and websites are notorious for "you-must-follow-these" training features and "run-these-miles-per-day" routines, but this is simply athletic entertainment. The more ambitious runners attempt to copy the latest big-city marathon winner's training habits—but most athletes can't duplicate these miles or paces (and professional athletes usually don't divulge their true schedules).

It is also common for runners to follow the workout schedules of their training partners or local running clubs, as social factors often replace physiology, logic, and individuality. Unfortunately, most runners fail to adhere to training schedules that best match their particular needs.

Barely a day goes by that I don't receive an email addressed to me at my website PhilMaffetone.com, which often begins as follows: "Dear Dr. Maffetone, I have just finished reading *The Big Book of Endurance Training and Racing* and I am planning to run a marathon next year, but I didn't find any specific training schedules to follow in your book . . ."

The reason that readers won't find one in that book, or in any of my books for that matter, is that all training needs to be individualized. This is true whether one is a 2:05 marathoner hoping to go even faster, or a competitive age-group runner trying to qualify for the Boston Marathon.

It is impossible to make training recommendations without knowing a runner's history, goals, physiology, his or her life's daily schedule, and conducting an in-person evaluation. With that said, in order to run a 1:59 marathon, our record-setting athlete will have to find his own optimal training routine.

The ideal schedule is not "one size fits all." Instead, it's an evolving, changing, living entity—one that a runner's personal well being should dictate from day to day. Even with the "perfect" schedule, there's really a range of training volume—a window that avoids overtraining and provides sufficient stimulation to get the most out of the body.

THE TRAINING SPECTRUM

The history of endurance training schedules has spanned the spectrum—from no workouts by competitors before the start of the 20th century, to high running mileage of greater intensity even before the running boom of the 1970s. Finding the balance between the extremes is important for the 1:59 marathoner if he is to fully develop his aerobic system, improve running economy and progress to 4:50 minutes-per-mile at the maximum aerobic heart rate in training. The actual weekly mileage required to reach this goal will certainly vary from one runner to the next.

Like Roger Bannister's light running schedule—twenty-five miles a week—in comparison to his competitors, the 1:59 marathoner might also dip below the current triple-digit-mile training tradition of elite runners to achieve superiority. Research continues to show that, in many cases, less training may be best.

High-mileage training weeks first became popular in the mid-1900s. The Finnish endurance runners of the first half of the 1900s may have been the first athletes to train with progressively more miles than was ever previously done. The trend is thought to have begun with Hannes Kolehmainen who won three gold medals while breaking two world records during the 1912 Olympic games. In 1920, Paavo Nurmi won three Olympic medals, then five more in the 1924 games, where Ville Ritola won four. Other Finns followed, including Volmari Iso-Hollo and Taisto Mäki. Years later, Lasse Viren soared as a Flying Finn at the 1972 and 1976 Olympics.

The high-mileage training trend has been copied ever since, especially here in the United States, despite the clear danger that it presents to runners who are unprepared to handle the physical stress, especially when combined with faster workouts. Both high volume and high intensity are the most common causes of overtraining, and in turn, this leads to chronic injuries.

Rather than use miles as your only training baseline, a much better factor to focus on is time. Only keeping track of miles can be misleading, and more is not always better. As aerobic function improves, the training pace quickens at the same heart rate. So a 5- or 10-mile run takes less time to complete. Instead of tracking miles, my recommended schedule would include the total time of each workout, including the weekly and monthly totals, all plotted out against pace. Rather than increasing quantity—the number of miles—the quality of each workout focuses on heart rate and time for the 1:59 marathoner. For example, an 8-mile run on Tuesday is a 45-minute workout. Rather than a 15-miler on Sunday, it's two hours.

WARMING UP AND COOLING DOWN

All training runs should begin with an active running warm-up and end with a cool-down. Yet when the topic of warming up is mentioned, many runners think of stretching. While stretching may be essential for those who participate in certain sports like track and field, gymnastics, and ballet, it does not produce a true warm-up and cool-down. Stretching is much less significant a need for endurance athletes, and it can even be harmful. A physically active warm-up and cool-down are ideal for runners—both don't require extremes in ranges of motion. A warm-up will also provide significant improvements in flexibility.

WARMING UP

One of the fastest ways to improve running economy is to properly warm up the body. Warming up refers to easy physical activity, usually slower running, that prepares the body for higher heart rate training.

A warm-up should be done before each workout, regardless of the type, and every race. Without it, bodily stress can affect muscles, joints, and other areas. A lack of warm-up can even stress the heart (as indicated by an electrocardiogram) due to reduced oxygenation of the heart muscle, and poor blood-pressure response following exercise, even in healthy, fit individuals.

After the first stage of the warm-up, which is a slight elevation of body temperature, a number of significant benefits occur, including:

- Increased blood flow to working muscles

- Increased oxygen availability

- Greater mechanical efficiency of joints, muscles, tendons, and ligaments

- Increased range of motion in joints

- Release of stored fat to be used for energy in aerobic muscles

- Increased breathing (lung) capacity

- Improved neuromuscular activity

In order to accomplish these positive changes, the muscle activity—the level of workout intensity—should begin very easy and gradually build up. Often, runners start their workouts too fast, not allowing for a proper warm-up, potentially causing physical stress.

A heart monitor is a helpful tool for warming up because it allows one to more accurately gauge the process. Let's use the example of a runner starting a one-hour aerobic workout with a maximum aerobic heart rate of 140 (with a range of 130–140). This athlete's starting heart rate is 60, so a proper warm-up means slowly running faster to gradually increase the HR to 140 over a period of at least fifteen minutes. The heart rate is slowly raised from the 60s to the 70s, 80s, and so forth until the 130–140 range is reached after fifteen minutes.

For training lasting more than about ninety minutes, the warm-up should be longer—perhaps about twenty minutes or more.

Ideally, the best warm-up is tailored to each runner's needs. Many individuals can feel the full-body benefit from better breathing, more flexibility and the loss of little aches or stiffness. Warming up is such a powerful tool it can even correct muscle imbalance.

Once you get used to warming up properly, and how it feels, you may notice your body requiring more warming, even for a short workout. If this is the case, extend your warm-up time. Never assume, however, that you need less than fifteen minutes, which seems to be the physiological minimum.

Cooling Down

An active cool-down refers to easy physical activity during the last part of your workout—just in the opposite order of the warm-up. The most important reason for a cool-down is that it begins a key process of recovery from the workout.

The cool-down slowly allows the heart rate to descend. While you will not reach your starting or resting heart rate, you may come within ten to twenty beats of it. Let's use the same example of the athlete above who began a run with a heart rate of 60 beats per minute and ascended to 140. Fifteen minutes before the end of the workout, the pace is reduced with the heart rate gradually diminished to 60 to 80 beats per minute.

This slow descent in intensity can help prevent physical and chemical stress, improving oxygenation and circulation in the muscles and removing blood lactate (even during an aerobic workout). These are all vital parts of the process of recovery.

For longer workouts, such as those of ninety minutes or two hours, increase the cool-down time to at least twenty minutes or more.

The time spent warming up and cooling down should be included as part of your total workout. So for a one-hour aerobic run, spend fifteen minutes warming up, fifteen cooling down, and a half hour in the maximum aerobic training zone.

Just because it doesn't feel like you're getting much of a workout during the warm-up and cool-down phases, they should still count as part of the overall training session. Tremendous health benefits are obtained through this component of training. A lack of warming up and cooling down can even contribute to overtraining.

LESS MAY BE BEST

The 1:59 marathoner may not need to have training runs much longer than two hours. In fact, a highly trained, well-rested, and healthy runner can perform a personal best with a regular long training run of less distance or time relative to the expected mileage or time of the race. But in this case, a two-hour run in the schedule, perhaps slightly longer to accommodate warming and cooling, will help ensure a well-developed aerobic system.

Fine-tuning one's workouts is accomplished to a great extent by continued evaluation. This will help the 1:59 marathoner, or any runner, find the most appropriate and balanced workout schedule. There might be some weeks, for example, when you are experiencing increased stress or deadlines in dealing with business issues, and you feel tired or fatigued at the start of your training runs. My recommendation is to reduce training, which will increase recovery and actually strengthen the body.

CATABOLIC AND ANABOLIC

Ask runners about their training schedules and you'll often hear long monologues about the miles they've logged, precise time of each run, or pace. But just focusing on these factors neglects a more significant component of optimal training. In fact, physiologically, the workout may be even less critical than another key part of the schedule that's often brushed aside and not emphasized—rest and recovery. The combination of one's run, and the recovery process, has to do with the body's catabolic, (associated with overreaching) and anabolic (recovery and rebuilding) balance.

Most endurance athletes have heard the terms catabolic and anabolic.

The catabolic response involves the many key changes that take place in the body during each run—it's the gas pedal you push down to get through the workout. This includes the normal physical wear and tear on muscles, ligaments, tendons, joints and bones. And it is associated with many chemical changes that occur in the body's complex metabolism, from the generation of additional energy, to increased circulation and respiration, and lactate regulation. This important training effect (when overreaching is optimal) results in a healthy tearing down of the body—and modifying it to create a better, stronger one, which is necessary, especially for a faster marathon.

All athletes experience the outcome of this catabolic state. It commonly includes relatively minor muscle or joints symptoms, such as mild achiness or weakness, and slight fatigue, all of which are more noticeable after a long workout. (Conversely, pain and exhaustion would indicate excessive wear and tear—a part of the overtraining syndrome.)

When the day's workout ends, another, perhaps more critical aspect of the schedule, is just beginning—anabolic activity. This is the time when the body rebuilds itself, so that the next bout of training can proceed with more efficiency and without harm, all while obtaining further benefits.

Anabolic is a term often associated with the illegal use of steroids (which, supposedly, helps speed recovery, allowing one to work out longer and harder, notwithstanding harmful side effects). But the body's natural catabolic and anabolic mechanisms are perfectly suited, in a healthy athlete, for the optimal training schedule. This catabolic-anabolic balance is the cycle of the athlete's life.

The anabolic aspect of the training schedule involves recovery; and this means getting sufficient rest. Unlike the catabolic gas pedal, the natural anabolic action is likened to the brakes that cause one to stop and take it easy. It allows the physical, chemical, and mental aspects of the body to revive themselves and fully heal. In fact, it's during this key anabolic recovery phase that the body gets stronger, faster, and builds more endurance.

This anabolic aspect of one's training schedule—the ability of the body to efficiently recover and rebuild following each day's workout—is as essential as the actual workout. Not only can it help propel the body towards greater athletic potential, but it can prevent injuries and illness as well.

A QUICK REVIEW

In the previous chapter, you were introduced to this formula:

Training = Workout + Rest

It is worth repeating here. Rest (or recovery) can be the secret to success for any runner and in particular, one seeking a 1:59 marathon because even a minor mishap in training is greatly amplified. One of the little known facts about why the Kenyans are the best distance runners of the modern era will surprise you. It's that they value their downtime. In addition to living and training at altitude, elite Kenyan runners spend a great deal of their day resting or sleeping when not training. Nap time is recovery time.

An optimal schedule is more than just monitoring miles or minutes—it balances the body's complex catabolic and anabolic features. And it can be demonstrated with the simple training formula.

Too much workout time (often from too many miles, too much intensity, or both), and not enough recovery (typically insufficient rest and sleep) cause an imbalanced training schedule, or overtraining. But even the easiest schedule can turn to overtraining if there is insufficient recovery to allow the body's anabolic rebuilding process to occur. This comes in the form of sleep, with virtually all adults requiring a minimum of about eight undisturbed hours each night (adolescents need much more). Some athletes may require additional sleep, but not less, prompting some to realize the benefits of a daytime nap. These should not last more than about an hour or they may interfere with your nighttime sleep routine.

WHAT YOU WON'T FIND IN THIS BOOK: SPECIFIC TRAINING PROGRAMS

There are probably any number of workout schedules that can prepare an elite runner for a 1:59 marathon, so long as the training equation stays balanced and the aerobic system continues to improve as indicated by a regular Maximum Aerobic Function

(MAF) Test. This will prevent excess training stress from disrupting the delicate equilibrium of the body's hormones, the neuromuscular system, proper brain chemistry, and the catabolic-anabolic balance, There is obviously no single running schedule to formulate a 1:59 marathon (or a 2:59 one), and if you've turned to this chapter in search of that special step-by-step program that will help you run a PR, it's simply not here. But the tools to create an individualized approach are present. They are detailed throughout this book, and by following these recommendations you truly have a golden opportunity to become a faster and more efficient runner.

For super-elite runners already on the cusp of making history, the road to a 1:59 marathon will still entail months of meticulous preparation. All other runners simply wanting to achieve new PRs also can benefit by being more attentive to the demands of scheduling and sticking to a game plan. Yet the plan needs to be flexible to allow for regular changes as the body adjusts and adapts in response to training. This means a schedule is always provisional, never followed blindly, but modified as often as the body demands it. Reading the body each day, taking measurements, is essential. If training appears comfortable, yet morning heart rate starts rising, MAF Test results diminish or symptoms such as fatigue, pain or other abnormal factors present themselves, it means training volume and/or intensity may be too much. The overall goal is to avoid injury, ill health, and other indications of impending overtraining. For example, if, on the morning after a two-hour run, your resting heart rate is ten beats higher than normal, this should alert you that the run might be too much at this point in the schedule. Or, if an MAF Test shows stagnating or slowing paces, you would want to further evaluate the cause of such a significant evaluation, before resuming more extensive training.

Finally, try not to be seduced by popular training trends. These include high-volume weeks, continuous track intervals, and hill repeats—separately or together, they can often impair the aerobic system and reduce running economy. Instead, consider these two training lessons:

- One's longest training run should only be two to two-and a-half hours in duration, including the warm-up and cool-down, with the rest at the maximum aerobic heart rate.
- As noted earlier, great marathons are run at a race pace that is *not* much above the maximum aerobic heart rate, such as 85 percent of one's VO_2max. So training above this level should be minimized or avoided.

FITNESS VS. HEALTH

When scheduling your training, it should be based on assessment, and the most critical factor here is that your health should *never* be compromised for increased fitness. Assessment-based training is individualized. If one runs ten hours each week, then ongoing evaluation will help determine if this is too much. If it is not, training volume may be increased slightly, following by further careful evaluations. This leads to fine-tuning a runner's program.

This process continues indefinitely. A marathoner must train hard enough, but avoid the pitfalls of overtraining, properly recover each day to avoid accumulating excess wear and tear, and maintain a healthy, fine-tuned body. This process is indicated not just by the absence of abnormal symptoms, but blood and other tests to ensure body chemistry supports the process, especially the MAF Test.

TRAINING TO FATIGUE

Another key feature of an optimal running schedule has to do with muscle fatigue. Virtually all runners know the feeling. It is more obvious in a race, when you want to keep going at the same pace but can't. The mind is willing but the body is tired and resisting. Power output cannot be maintained. While fatigue is expected during a race, this should not be the case during aerobic training. There is, however, a certain level of normal muscle fatigue with training, especially during overreaching. But too much fatigue is abnormal, can impair progress, reduce health, and ultimately ruin your upcoming race.

In a clinic or laboratory, muscle fatigue can be measured in a single muscle or group as a reduction of power. In the case of the entire body, sufficient fatigue reduces the pace at the maximum aerobic heart rate. This will be evident in one's MAF Test.

Mild and moderate muscle fatigue is normal and even necessary during a balanced training schedule. It is part of the overreaching process, ultimately helping the body accomplish more work with the same effort. This results in faster running at the same heart rate— improved running economy.

While normal, healthy fatigue encourages muscles to adapt and prepare for additional power, there are other benefits. These include the following: improved heart, circulation, and lung function, enhanced regulation of oxygen and carbon dioxide, better utilization of muscle energy, and optimal metabolism of lactate.

Problems arise when the delicate balance of training and recovery is disturbed. Too much intensity or higher volume training can cause undue, *excessive* muscle fatigue. This leads to the first stage of overtraining, when muscles are abnormally damaged. The body has built a "debt" of muscle fatigue, whereby training exceeds the ability to properly recover. It can eventually trigger muscle imbalance and injury, and impair the aerobic system. Just a single "over-fatiguing" session can cause damage, especially without appropriate recovery. The runner may pay the penalty of poor performance on race day because muscle fatigue still exists. (The same challenge exists when racing too frequently.)

Excess fatigue is often glorified in the "no pain, no gain" training ethic. While some athletes, such as those in track and field, powerlifting, and football, get closer to the line of overtraining and are injured more easily, runners are much different. Running relies mostly on aerobic training, which, when done properly, does not produce excess muscle fatigue unless the *volume* of training is excessive.

Here are some factors associated with excess muscle fatigue:

- Fatigue generated by an intense workout can increase the stress hormone cortisol and potentially impair the aerobic system.
- A muscle that is fatigued will not contract as many fibers, reducing power and increasing weakness.
- Muscle fatigue can affect associated joint movements (for example, quadriceps and knee joint), and contribute to such chronic conditions as osteoarthritis.
- Poor posture and gait irregularity result from excess muscle fatigue. This problem can last many hours or days following training, and require more recovery.
- Working a fatigued muscle can lead to muscular imbalance and result in further damage to ligaments, tendons, joints, fascia, or bone.
- A fatigue-producing anaerobic interval track workout, like a popular weight lifting session, can require significant

recovery—at least 48 hours, often more, before working out again.

- Excess muscle fatigue can significantly reduce training and racing performance.
- During competition, varying one's speed can cause more muscle fatigue compared to racing at a steady-state pace.
- Respiratory (breathing) muscles can often fatigue, sometimes more than leg muscles, and limit maximum exercise intensity and duration.
- Poor body balance can result in muscle fatigue, and lead to inefficient joint movement.
- Muscle fatigue can worsen symptoms of pain (and also chronic fatigue syndrome and fibromyalgia).
- Anaerobic-muscle fibers fatigue much more easily and quickly than aerobic ones.
- Excess muscle fatigue can quickly worsen running economy.

While training, excess muscle fatigue usually only occurs when running above the maximum aerobic heart rate. The exception may include if the runs are too long, or the increase in training volume occurs too quickly.

THE TRAINING TAPER

A proper taper is a useful approach to keep fatigue in check before race day arrives. But it is equally important to include tapering within the boundaries of one's training schedule. This is especially true before long runs of, say, two hours. Among other things, it helps ensure recovery.

A training taper involves a reduction in workouts (volume and intensity), for a day or two previous to a long run. The benefits include higher quality workouts, faster pace, and better overall training effect.

A taper is also valuable at the conclusion of a long aerobic training period and the start of the racing season. While a taper leading up to a marathon might begin two weeks before the race, training tapers can be short, such as scheduling easier days of running and sometimes a day off before a two-hour run.

When tapering for a marathon, reduce training in a stepwise fashion by 50 to 70 percent with less running as race day approaches. Add some off days during this period. For example, in a two-week taper, take one or two days off each week, including a day or two before the race. Easy walking workouts of thirty minutes can be used during these "off" days to keep your body loose and warmed up.

Tapering does not result in lost fitness. In fact, your muscle strength can actually increase and there should be no reduction in your MAF Test results. Tapering is not the same as detraining, which is the complete cessation of workouts. With zero training, endurance is adversely affected within a two-week period. Even though the taper period is 50 to 70 percent less training, your fitness level is maintained; in fact, it can improve because recovery accelerates.. A proper pre-race taper can also improve running economy.

100-PLUS MILE WEEKS: JUST HOW NECESSARY?

For elite runners, learning to optimize their training schedule requires the ability to combine art and science, trial and error, intuition, and maybe even some good fortune. Yet too often, the one missing element is rest. More mileage and faster workouts don't always produce positive results when the body isn't adequately rested or prepared to handle the accumulated stress.

"You feel like if you're taking time off you didn't really earn it," Ryan Hall told *Sports Illustrated* in a 2012 interview. "But if you come out of a rested state, you perform better. After having trained so hard for so long and looking at other athletes, thinking, `I trained 10 times harder than these guys and they're killing me in races,' you learn that more is not always better."

Then how do runners know when they find themselves on the dangerous slippery slope of overtraining? One of the first signs is too many miles. (Ultrarunning is different since the pace is slower.) The obsession with hitting or surpassing 100 miles each week wrongly convinces many runners that they have achieved something special, that they are following in the footsteps of say, Bill Rodgers, who often averaged 150-mile weeks by usually running twelve miles in the morning and twelve miles later in the day.

The notion that running over 100 miles every week is a baseline for fast marathon times is misleading since it doesn't take into account the more critical factor of time. For elite runners, a century week might mean sixteen hours of weekly training, and for another thirteen, and still another eighteen. But the real problem with this much running, in addition to significantly increasing the need for recovery, is scheduling and training twice daily like Rodgers did (and popularized) all those years when he was winning the Boston and New York City Marathons. How else can one run 100, 150, or more miles in a single week without doubling up on workouts for several days?

The two-runs-a-day training schedule remains popular among today's top runners, and it can have significant benefits, but only when properly applied. Double-daily runs can encourage the body to work more efficiently under a moderate level of fatigue, and may help speed recovery. Top Kenyan runners, for example, are well known for their two-a-days. But when they are not training, they are sleeping and resting.

Two-a-day workouts require additional recovery time because of the added training stress. But this approach does *not* require two runs for several days a week. A better method is scheduling a single day of two runs, followed by another workout the next morning. Two-a-days only work in a healthy body.

Once you can get past the "more is better" temptation, it is best to replace it with "less is best." Of the thousands of runners who initially consulted with me during my coaching career, hardly any were undertrained, and the majority ran too many miles. I often found myself reducing a runner's workout schedule by 15, 20 or even 30 percent. As a result, their race times would drop with decreased training.

A BALANCED SCHEDULE

This brings me to the importance of creating a balanced weekly schedule. A healthy and safe way to accomplish it is to emphasize three key days. One is an off-day, another a double workout, and a third is the long day.

- Off-days are required whenever you feel the need arise. For most runners, "when in doubt, rest" usually works well because their brains are telling them something critical. In addition, off-days should become a weekly feature, especially in the period leading up to big races. These are best placed before or after a long or double day, or as part of a taper for a race. Off-days should further complement regular rests—nightly sleeping of eight hours, and even a nap if needed.

- Double days involve two runs within about twelve hours, followed by another the next morning. You can perform two training runs on the first day, one morning and a second later in the day—as far apart from each other as possible. This day is followed by another run the next morning, one that is shorter, giving the body three workouts in a relatively short period of time. This strategy, performed only once per week, can help train the body by carefully pushing one into overreaching, and can encourage the body to recover faster. However, it works only if the athlete maintains adequate rest.

- The long day is when you train for the most hours. For marathoners, this should not be more than two and a half hours (including warm-up and cool-down), especially since it is best to spend about two hours running at one's maximum aerobic heart rate (or at least perform aerobic intervals). This day is best preceded by an off or easier short-run day, so the body is better rested going into the workout. And, it is followed the next day by a very easy and shorter run, later in the same day if possible, to allow extra recovery time. Additionally, long runs are best performed in the morning.

Here is an example of a balanced weekly schedule:

Mon	Tues	Wed	Thurs	Fri	Sat	Sun
30-45 min (pm)	60-90 min	60 min	45 min 60 min (pm)	60 min	off	2+hr

For those unable to have this much time to train, this approach may be too stressful. But for elites with more training and recovery time available, some of these runs can be increased—but only as a gradual buildup.

Our 1:59 marathoner won't be someone who has run his body into the ground with overtraining. Instead, he will have smartly balanced all the necessary diet, training and lifestyle factors. The training schedule should work in tandem with regular assessments. As training and recovery continue to progress, testing the body to guarantee that all is well should remain an integral part of overall conditioning. This will help avoid drifting past the overreaching state into the red zone of overtraining. Properly monitoring the day-to-day workout and health status helps to ensure that one is achieving adequate training stimulation while avoiding overtraining. It's how our 1:59 marathoner will prove to the world that the human body can break the two-hour barrier. For all other runners, who want to set new PRs, the same lessons certainly apply.

CHAPTER 8
MUSCLE BALANCE

Lasse Viren, who I worked with in Finland, when he took his shirt off, he looked like a plucked chicken. There is no muscle at all, just ribs sticking out. He won four Olympic Gold Medals!

—ARTHUR LYDIARD

We all know that the world's top distance runners are exceptionally lean. These endurance athletes have little body fat, but they also don't have much muscle mass either. Yet it's those same muscles, when sufficiently strong, that can help carry a marathoner to a 1:59 historic finish.

To understand why, we need to look at muscles in a different light—and not one commonly associated with power and strength activities such as weightlifting, bodybuilding, and CrossFit. Muscle activity is the combination of contraction and relaxation, actions controlled by the brain. Our muscles maintain posture, hold up the skeleton, guide our every motion, and allow us to walk and run. When the muscles work well, running economy can be significantly improved.

Muscles do more than physically move and support us. Equally important for training and racing, as well as for good health, is their chemical activity. These include the generation of energy (from fat and sugar), immune activity (helping recover from workout and races), and the production of hormones (myokines, the chemicals released with muscle contraction that communicate with the rest of the body).

This chapter highlights two key physical issues associated with optimal muscle movement. First is muscle balance. This involves the ideal amount of contraction and relaxation for each step one takes in every workout and race. The second is strength, something most marathoners have too little of, despite their endurance.

Muscle Balance

Muscle balance is really about two primary ideas. First, muscles work together. In order for balance to exist, the brain must coordinate the right combination of contraction and relaxation with each stride of a training run or race. In fact, running relies on more of the body's muscles than almost all other activities. Not just in the legs, but throughout the whole body, from head to toe. All of the muscles must work together in harmony to create the fluid motion we so often observe in top marathoners. Balanced muscles promote improved economy.

The second notion is that two or more muscles can develop an imbalance. This is sometimes obvious, such as a runner who might slightly favor one side, even limp, or make movements that don't create a nice fluid gait. But often, a silent and somewhat subtle muscle imbalance exists that is less noticeable. This is not as easily observed, but it can definitely reduce running economy.

Many runners are able to sense subtle changes when their running seems not quite right. But when they are asked, "What's wrong?" their answers tend to be vague. Typical replies are: "Something is just not right" or "my stride feels off." Usually, the cause is some type of muscle imbalance.

Let's now look more closely at normal muscle movement and its to-be-avoided counterpart, muscle imbalance.

Muscles typically work together during activity—one tightens or contracts to perform a specific action, while another, often on the opposite side of an arm or leg, relaxes. In fact, in order for one muscle to contract, its opposing muscle must first relax. It's easy to feel a muscle contract, but the one relaxing initially is not easily detectable.

As one runs, this same contraction and relaxation takes place constantly in opposing muscles. It occurs in the quadriceps (front of the thigh) and hamstrings (back of the thigh), the anterior tibialis muscle (front of the leg) and calf muscles (including the gastrocnemius and posterior tibialis), the pectoralis muscles (upper chest and front shoulder) and latissimus (back of shoulder and spine), and so on.

When you lift the knee while running, it is because the quadriceps muscles contract. But before that can happen, the hamstrings must first relax. Without this relaxation-contraction occurring effectively, such as when one muscle relaxes too much or another contracts too much, there's muscle imbalance.

Using the knee-lifting example, when you contracted the quads the hamstrings first relaxed. Now imagine if the quads remained tight and the hamstrings remained too relaxed, even when you're not running. In this situation, you might experience a feeling of tightness in your quad. Or, lifting your knee up and down might not feel quite right, with discomfort or even pain. This is a state of muscle imbalance, which also involves the nerves connecting the motor area of the brain to the muscles (the *neuromuscular system*).

With muscle imbalance, the muscle that stays overly relaxed is too loose (referred to as *abnormal inhibition*) and sometimes called "weak" (although this is not true weakness, which refers to the lack of power). In most cases, this looseness affects a second, opposite muscle to become too tight. Meanwhile, muscle tightness (called *abnormal facilitation*) is sometimes called spasm (but technically not an accurate term for most cases).

113

Muscle imbalance can adversely affect many body areas. This includes the joint(s) they move, the tendons they're attached to, and other muscles, ligaments, fascia, bones, and body structures (such as the pelvis, spine, or head). The result is often a body-wide irregularity in posture and gait—a reason it can significantly affect running economy.

Muscle imbalance can be relatively minor, causing minimal impairment, or in some cases extreme to the point of causing severe pain in a joint controlled by that muscle.

The development of muscle imbalance usually starts with a muscle that's too relaxed, loose or "weak"—for various reasons it becomes abnormally lengthened, overstretched or "pulled." In some cases this muscle problem is silent. However, you might feel the lack of function produced by it, such as sensing something not right in the knee joint while running or experiencing low back pain after a race.

The tight side of muscle imbalance is typically uncomfortable and sometimes painful. Tight muscles are shortened, a reason stretching was so popular (and should be avoided); however, in most cases, this would be not be treating the cause of the imbalance which is usually the loose muscle. In attempting to loosen a tight muscle through stretching, you can actually worsen the loose one even more by stretching it further. My recommendation: Don't stretch!

In addition, an imbalanced pair of muscles in one body area could affect others. This *domino effect* is a clinical pattern commonly found in athletes—one muscle problem affects another, and so on, with the first few being silent but then ending with intense pain in a particular body area. This is how a muscle imbalance in the foot, for example, can alter the lower back, or a certain neck muscle impairment adversely alters proper trunk rotation while running.

Common Causes of Muscle Imbalance

Here are some of the most common causes of muscle imbalance.

1. Improper Training. This can arise from a disruption in the training equation (training = workout + rest), such as too much running and insufficient rest or recovery. Interval or other anaerobic workouts cause muscle imbalance much easier than aerobic training due to the added stress.

2. Improper Running Shoes. Footwear that is over-supportive, too small, with an outsized heel, extra cushioning, or has a narrow toe box, can all lead to muscle imbalance—and not just in your legs.

3. Local Injury. Common muscle strains can be due to over-stretching, overstriding, or a twisted ankle on a trail.

4. Nutritional Factors. These may include low dietary protein, dehydration, anemia, low blood sugar, and poor nutrition such as inadequate caloric intake.

5. Pain. Whether from unknown sources, chronic or acute pain from an injury or illness, the presence of pain itself can produce muscle imbalance, and worse, it can create a vicious cycle of cause and effect.

6. The use of non-steroidal anti-inflammatory drugs (NSAIDs) can also cause muscle imbalance, especially when taken before, during or after a race or training run. These include aspirin, ibuprofen, Advil, Motrin, Nuprin, Naprosyn, and other prescription and over-the-counter drugs.

7. Chronic Illness. These include diabetes, sarcopenia (reduced muscle bulk with aging or protein deficient diet), chronic inflammation,

arthritis, heart disease, and various neurological disorders such as Parkinson's disease, stroke, and spinal cord injuries.

SELF-CARE

When muscle imbalance causes pain or dysfunction to persist and interfere with training and racing, treatment by a health professional may be necessary. But many runners are able to correct their own imbalances using the following home remedies:

- First is to address the cause or causes of muscle imbalance as discussed above.
- A *healthy* body will often correct itself. This is especially true in those who have a well-functioning aerobic system. In particular, the process of a good, slow warm-up before a run can often correct muscle imbalance.
- Barefoot therapy can correct muscle imbalance (discussed in the next chapter).
- The application of cold (cryotherapy) can help correct muscle imbalance. But continued use of ice placed directly against the body, or a body part plunged into a freezing ice bath may cause muscle damage. A cold wet towel kept in the refrigerator and placed on the body for 10 minutes several times daily can be very effective. (Heat usually won't correct muscle imbalance and may even aggravate it.)

Another cause of muscle imbalance may be due to lifting weights incorrectly. An example is trying to strengthen the quadriceps on a weight machine without properly and proportionately doing the same for the hamstrings. This is a daunting task for anyone to attempt.

Fortunately, there are easy, safe and effective ways for a runner to improve strength.

STRENGTH TRAINING

Endurance is obviously a key part of training for a 1:59 marathon. It involves building the aerobic system while avoiding too much anaerobic and other stress factors. However, strength, especially in the lower limb muscles is vital for strong marathon performances, and another necessary training component. Compared to building a healthy aerobic system, strength may play a lesser role in the marathon—but still enough of a factor to allow some of today's top distance runners to inch their way down to 1:59. That's because stronger muscles can improve running economy.

One problem that many runners share is a hidden, body-wide weakness in muscles, despite possessing terrific endurance. Technically, it's muscular strength that is low. It's easy to demonstrate when the right health professional performs muscle testing or uses various types of electronic or other technologies that measure muscle power. But a simple indication of weakness can be found with a standard test of jumping ability that any runner can do (see sidebar on page 119).

Ask a group of marathoners to perform the standing vertical jump test and most usually won't get higher than twelve inches or so, well below the athletic average and significantly lower than sprinters and middle-distance runners. In fact, most sprinters can jump vertically well into the twenty-inch range and beyond. That's because in many cases, the marathoner's lower body muscles have too little strength. In making the transition from 5K and 10K speed, many marathoners lose that strength. This may be due to overtraining, frequent muscle fatigue, or a dwindling strength loss in those approaching age thirty.

But successful training for a 1:59 marathon will require getting a modest amount of this strength back.

Correcting the problem of low muscle strength can improve marathon times for all runners, because it can help running economy. In particular, *proper* strength training can allow the muscles to utilize more *elastic energy* and reduce the amount of energy wasted when the foot hits the ground (discussed in the following chapter). The improved running economy may be the result of improvements in the neuromuscular system, which can increase the number of muscle fibers that contract in each muscle.

All of this poses a potentially challenging task; How can a runner incorporate strength training without increasing bulk and body weight, risking injury or overtraining, impairing endurance, and fatiguing muscles excessively? Here is a marathoner's wish list when it comes to strength training:

- Improve strength *and* endurance at the same time.
- Short, easy, and non-tiring exercises that still increase strength.
- Bones must also get stronger as they are the foundational support of muscular attachments.
- Workouts must not interfere with aerobic progress by causing undue stress such as raising cortisol levels.
- Strength workouts must not require additional recovery time in the training schedule.
- The workouts should not cause excess muscle fatigue.
- Weight workouts should not place a runner at high risk for injury.

Strength training won't improve VO_2max or lactate threshold in well-trained runners. That's not the goal. But studies have shown that strength training can help running economy by 8 percent, which is a significant increase. Furthermore, it is best to strengthen the entire body

THE VERTICAL JUMP TEST

This is easiest in the presence of another person helping to mark your jump height.

- While standing next to a wall flatfooted and barefoot, reach your arm up as high as possible and mark the wall (or place a piece of tape) at the highest point of your fingertips.
- Stand in the same location next to the wall, and jump up as high as possible and make a second mark on the wall at your highest point (or place a piece of tape). Be sure to bend the knees well before jumping to obtain the best possible results.
- Perform three tests and record the highest jump by measuring the difference between the low and high mark on the wall. This is your vertical jump height.

Perform this test every month or two throughout the year to make sure improvements are being realized.

rather than individual muscles by the addition of weight. This allows gravity to trigger both the muscles *and* bones to become stronger.

Mention strength training and many runners think of the following: tough hill repeats, interval workouts, or other anaerobic runs. But these workouts don't produce the near-maximum muscle contractions that can increase strength like the correct weight program. And, as previously mentioned, anaerobic training can have a negative impact on building an effective aerobic system.

Many runners incorporate traditional weight-lifting programs in their regular training. This might involve going to the gym several times a week. Once there, they go from one machine to the next, using higher reps and lower weights. But this type of approach can be a disaster for a runner's aerobic system and negatively impact one's marathon performance. The reasons have to do with muscle bulk, which can add significant body weight, the production of excess muscle fatigue, which can interfere with one's gait, and the release of stress hormones adversely affecting the aerobic system. These problems can significantly lead to reductions in running economy.

An example of the stress associated with traditional weight workouts is the usual requirement of a forty-eight-hour recovery time. This is due to excess muscle fatigue and associated stress hormone responses. But even performing an easy training run within this forty-eight-hour window can add to an already stressful condition, with the real potential of impairing the aerobic system and pushing one toward overtraining. Some studies show that adequate recovery from traditional weight training could take *more than* forty-eight hours. This type of routine, which includes a high number of reps, little rest between sets and lifting to fatigue, should be avoided.

For runners, strength goals should address the improvement of the whole body without impairing endurance, and be able to continue training the same or next day without pain, fatigue, or the risk of overtraining. This can be accomplished with the following:

- The use of relatively heavy weights
- Fewer repetitions
- Not lifting to fatigue
- Resting three minutes between sets

Strength is not always associated with muscle size. The brain plays a significant role in how much power a muscle generates, stimulating nerves that innervate individual muscle fibers to contract. The more fibers contracted, the more strength. Just having a large mass of muscle does not assure more fibers will be stimulated to generate extra power. A very lean athlete who can contract a lot of muscle fibers can be stronger than a bulky athlete who can't contract as many fibers.

A muscle that is fatigued won't contract as many fibers either. So it's important to avoid workouts that are performed to more than mild fatigue. Avoid what is often encouraged in the gym—lifting to significant fatigue, sometimes to exhaustion.

This is not to say your muscles won't get a bit tired when working out properly, just like after a long run. But it's critical to avoid significant fatigue, which can be felt the next day as muscle soreness or even pain.

Despite the hype found in many magazine articles and on websites, not all weight-training routines result in better bone strength. In fact, the "no pain, no gain" approach can sometimes reduce overall bone strength, not to mention increase the risk of overtraining and injury.

Runners can take a valuable lesson from Olympic weightlifters. These power athletes want the most strength they can get from their bodies but with the least amount of muscle weight gain, since this would put them into a higher weight category where competition may be more difficult. Apart from the heavyweight and super-heavyweight categories, these athletes are generally not bulky, but have very strong muscles and bones—more so than bodybuilders who tend to be bulkier and not as strong.

Lifting heavier weight with fewer repetitions, and more rest between sets, increases muscle strength and bone density better than lifting lighter weights with higher repetitions and less rest. This does not mean more weight is better. To avoid fatigue, overtraining, or causing an acute injury, the amount of weight that might be appropriate is about 80 percent of your one-repetition maximum weight. This is also the weight you can lift about six times *before* fatigue develops.

The strength-training plan should be simple and safe. You really only need to perform a couple of routines per workout to build whole-body muscle and bone strength, and without interfering with your aerobic system. The two easiest and most effective ones include the deadlift and squat (front, overhead, and/or back). Here are some examples:

- Reps: 1–6 reps in each set
- Sets: 4 (more if time and energy permit)
- Lifting should be done relatively fast, not slow
- Recovery between sets should be three minutes (timed), more if desired
- All movements should be smooth and natural
- As you get stronger, slowly increase the amount of weight rather than repetitions
- Three times per week, more if time permits

Here is a sample of a specific workout:

- Warm up: 15 minutes (walk, easy run or other aerobic activity)
- Deadlift: 5 reps
- Recovery: 3 minutes

- Squat: 5 reps
- Recovery: 3 minutes
- Repeat above lifts three more times
- Cool down (same as warm-up)

When starting a strength program, begin with less weight and fewer reps—and be very conservative. Take several weeks to increase weight and reps. In many cases, use a plain barbell without any extra weight so you get used to the movements, then slowly add small amounts of weight every couple of weeks.

If you're new to lifting weights, I recommend getting some one-on-one guidance from a trained professional who can help you with technique.

WEIGHT WARM-UP

A warm-up for a weight workout is simple. Here are two options. Perform strength training immediately following a short or medium aerobic run, of say, an hour or less. Or, walk for fifteen minutes as

SLOW WEIGHTS: THE EFFECTIVE STAY-AT-HOME WORKOUT

Many runners have specified periods of time during the day or evening for strength training, which includes the routine of changing clothes and driving to a nearby gym. None of this may be necessary.

Instead, you can do the weight workout as part of your day, just like you do other chores or activities such as cooking or checking email. Because you're only taking a few seconds or minutes for each set—lifting a weight six times or less—then going about your other business until you can do another set, you won't sweat, get out of breath or need to sit and rest. How long you wait between sets is not important, so long as the time gap is at least three minutes. But it can be an hour or two, or more.

All you will need in terms of equipment is a simple set of weights, including barbells and/or dumbbells.

The end-result of slow weights is the same as if you went to the gym, but without the time and cost. Slow weights will strengthen your muscles and bones, but won't build muscle bulk and lead to weight gain. And, unlike most weight training, this routine won't interfere with aerobic function.

For many runners, slow weights can be their regular strength training routine—by not tacking on another workout to an already busy schedule, it may mean more time for recovery.

But when performing slow weights, like all other healthy workouts, don't forget to bring your brain along. For example, don't finish a stressful business phone call, then go to your weights and try to "iron out" your frustrations. Instead, when you hit the home weights, close your eyes, breathe, relax, and be in the moment—focus on what you're about to do, then do it.

For some people, performing slow weights during daytime hours might be difficult. Work schedules may not allow it. Although in many other cases, two small dumbbells on the floor in a nearby corner in your home office or bedroom is a convenient possibility, even if they are only used during the evening hours.

The bottom line is that, for most runners, perhaps two, three or more times during the seven-day week, slow weights can successfully be incorporated into the day or evening schedule. As little as two exercises of up to six reps and three sets, for example, would provide a significant workout.

Perform slow weights throughout the day and/or evening and you will have accomplished an effective workout. Don't be fooled by the apparent simplicity, or the fact that your muscles won't feel sore.

Lift about one rep every second or two—but taking time between sets, which is minimally three, but may be five or ten minutes, or a half hour or more. Even go two or more hours between sets depending on the day's schedule as the effects are cumulative.

A typical slow weight weekly workout may include lifting three or four days (although five or six is fine too); each lift is about 80 percent of the maximum weight one can lift one time for that exercise; three to four sets each day, or more; up to six repetitions per set; resting between sets is at least three minutes, but an hour or two or more is perfectly fine.

If you're new to strength training, make sure that you are conservative in all aspects of slow weights, just like other exercise routines. Once you ramp up with regular workouts of three days a week or more, and get stronger, you can perform slow weights everyday if you want. Properly done, it won't produce any significant soreness because you're recovering after each set throughout the workout. And because of this, and you're not lifting to fatigue or exhaustion, you don't build bulk but strengthen both bones and muscles. As strength increases, add more weight rather than more reps or sets.

I would not recommend slow weights first thing in the morning. It's best that you warm up your body first. Also avoid doing slow weights right after a long run or an anaerobic workout, since you'll need that time and energy for recovery.

a warm-up before the strength workout. Either way, a properly executed warm up should be part of every workout.

For many runners, following a program that I call *slow weights* can make building more muscle and bone strength just as effective and less time-consuming than going to the gym.

DANGERS OF STRETCHING

Stretching muscles does not accomplish what a real warm-up does. Nor will it prevent injury or improve performance. Instead, it can have the opposite effect—stretching can be harmful.

It's critical that runners increase their *flexibility*. But this can be done just as effectively, and without risk of injury, with a proper warm-up.

Generally, runners who stretch are injured more frequently than those who don't stretch. That has not only been my observation over the past thirty-five years, but the opinion and observation of many other healthcare professionals, and has been well documented by scientific studies.

There are two basic types of stretching, static and ballistic. Static stretching is a slow, deliberate movement, in which you lightly stretch a muscle and hold it statically for ten to thirty seconds. When properly done, this activity promotes relaxation of the muscle being stretched. Optimal static stretching requires that each muscle group be sequentially repeated three to four times. It also demands that the activity be done slowly and not rushed. Static stretching can be done actively or passively. Of these, active is much safer than passive.

- Active stretching is accomplished by contracting the antagonist muscle (the one opposite the muscle you're stretching). For example, to actively stretch the hamstring muscles, the quadriceps muscles are contracted.

• Passive stretching uses gravity or force from another body part or person to move a body segment to the end of its range of motion or beyond—the reason this form of stretching can so easily cause injury.

The second basic type of stretching is called ballistic. This is a "bouncing" method and is the most common type of stretching done by athletes. It makes use of the body's momentum to repeatedly stretch a joint position to or beyond the extreme ranges of motion. Because this method is more rapid than static stretching, it activates the stretch reflex, which increases tension in the muscle, rather than relaxation. This can result in micro-tearing of muscle fibers with resultant injury.

Look around before the start of a marathon and it is not unusual to see many runners performing ballistic stretching. Pre-race tension tends to make nervous runners stretch in a quick, and hence more ballistic mode. Likewise before a training run—most runners are in a hurry and end up performing ballistic stretches. This should be avoided at all costs.

THE FLEXIBILITY FACTOR AND YOGA

Flexibility refers to the relative range of motion allowed by the muscles around a joint. This is related to the tension in the muscles that move or restrict the joint. Muscle balance may be the most important aspect of flexibility, with muscle imbalance producing reduced flexibility in a given joint. Overall, a healthy, warmed-up body is more flexible.

Aerobic function improves flexibility because of its effect on muscle function. Those with a greater aerobic system generally have more flexibility—not too much or too little. Those with too much flexibility also risk injury as the muscles allow joints to move too far from their normal ranges of motion.

It should be noted that yoga and other "whole-body" flexibility activities are quite different from stretching as I've described it above. When properly performed using a very slow, deliberate, and easy motion, whole-body flexibility activities are healthy, safe, and effective. However, most runners who I've observed doing yoga, Pilates, or other activities to improve flexibility, do them improperly—too fast and too hard. In addition, since these activities don't provide a sufficient warm-up, an active warm-up should precede them—such as performing yoga after an aerobic run.

Slow weights offer the option of performing strength workouts whenever the time and energy allows it. In some ways, it is like an indoor *fartlek* workout with weights. For others, a more structured strength-training program, properly executed, can be just as effective. However one accomplishes better muscular strength, improved running economy will follow.

MUSCLE MYSTERY

There are many elite marathoners who are capable of running 2:10 or faster. Not only do they possess high VO_2max and lactate thresholds, they are also potential candidates to race 1:59, especially if they improve the efficiency of their muscle function. Even relatively small changes can have a dramatic effect in boosting running economy. With better muscle mechanics, a runner's gait becomes more fluid, and each footstrike is better able to convert gravity stress into useable energy via elastic recoil. There is also an overall reduction in body-wide wear-and-tear with each mile run over the course of the marathon. This also impacts brain function, which does not have to compensate for physical imbalances throughout the body.

Yet, muscles and their influence on running economy are still a mystery to exercise and gait researchers in the laboratory. While scientists might measure a single muscle group's power, along with fiber types, contractile features, endurance components, and other important features, the bigger picture is still missing—how can our muscles actually improve economy and make us run faster?

The gap between the academic world and real world of coaches and athletes remains wide. Despite its obvious importance, the practical aspect of the full spectrum of our neuromuscular system is somewhat lacking, and it's the primary reason that running economy is still not well understood. Instead, researchers—and those in the media who try translating this textbook information to the running public—zero in on such things as VO_2max, lactate, and anaerobic threshold notions, which, as important as they may be, are less relevant for a sub-two-hour marathon.

As many elite runners already know firsthand, the regular use of physical trainers, massage therapists, and sports medicine expert can help improve muscle balance and strength, and potentially lead to better running economy. These practitioners have a variety of hands-on techniques in their wellness toolkit. Successful results often occur with measureable changes in posture, gait, strength and the ability to run faster at the same heart rate. While the outcomes of these approaches are clear, just how exactly they work is much more fuzzy.

Unfortunately, there are many treatment methods that might subjectively feel good to the runner, such as relieving a muscle ache here, correcting a tendon tweak there, but they don't always produce measureable improvements over time. One reason for this is a reliance on a "cookbook" therapeutic approach that is symptom-based. What should be emphasized instead is a holistic (big picture) understanding that considers all aspects of the individual runner—training schedules, nutrition, stress issues—since any or all of these can have impact on muscle function. The nature of this approach, in which each runner is treated individually, is not one well suited to laboratory testing.

There are plenty of therapists who have deviated from the symptom-oriented therapy approach that modern healthcare now demands. They are found among the many sports specialties, including physical therapy, kinesiology, biofeedback, chiropractic, massage therapy, as well as some medical doctors and osteopaths. These holistic-minded therapists employ posture and gait evaluation, muscle testing, blood and other lab tests, and dietary analysis that are important for improving both health and fitness. They include the ability to assess and correct imbalances beginning with the first therapy session, then use all running factors reflected by the muscles—including gait, strength, heart rate, and pace—to help guide training effectiveness and avoid overtraining and prevent injury. For elite as well as recreational runners, the most difficult part is finding the right therapist. There is no doubt that the 1:59 marathon runner will be working with a therapist—or even more than one. Going 1:59 will ultimately be a team effort.

CHAPTER 9

FEET FIRST

Shoes do no more for the foot than a hat does for the brain.
—DR. MERCER RANG, legendary orthopedic surgeon and
researcher in pediatric development

Will our first 1:59 marathoner be wearing racing flats? Or will he be running barefoot?

Over 50 years ago, Ethiopia's Abebe Bikila raced barefoot to Olympic marathon victory on Rome's asphalt roads, including a stretch of cobblestones along the Appian Way. Bikila had been a last-minute addition to the Ethiopian team, replacing an injured teammate. Runners were supposed to race in Adidas shoes—the German footwear company was the Games' sponsor—but Bikila found none that fit comfortably. So he decided to run without shoes.

Going barefoot made perfect sense for the lean, taller-than-average Ethiopian, who was born in the small village of Jato. He led an active childhood as a shepherd for his father's flock. In his late teens, he joined the army's imperial bodyguard regiment where his natural running talents emerged during mandatory fitness events among the military services.

In his first annual National Army Athletic competition at the age of twenty-eight, he finished the marathon in 2:39:50. This impressive showing by a running novice caught the attention of Swedish coach Onni Niskanen, who was then director of athletics under the ministry of education and later an official of the Red Cross. Under Niskanen's guidance, Bikila focused his energy on marathon-specific training for the 1960 Olympics.

Once in Rome, Bikila lined up at the marathon start with sixty-seven of the world's fastest distance runners. Many wore colors of the countries that were distance-running powerhouses at the time—Ireland, Great Britain, New Zealand, Australia, and Morocco. Some of Bikila's fellow racers probably shook their heads at the sight of this unknown marathoner, an alternate, and who wasn't even wearing shoes! But Bikila proved that he was there to win, comfortably staying mid-pack during the first half of the race before pulling away with several other runners. With one kilometer left, Bikila turned on his barefoot jets, his feet rhythmically slapping the pavement, and finished the race in a record time of 2:15:16, beating the one set at the 1952 Helsinki Games by about eight minutes.

Reporters swarmed around Bikila at the finish, demanding to know why he ran without shoes. His reply seemed less about himself and more about the pride that he felt about his homeland: "I wanted the whole world to know that my country, Ethiopia, has always won with determination and heroism."

A hero to millions worldwide and the first black African to win a gold medal in the Olympics, Bikila still felt the sting of racism when a British sports magazine wrote, "[Rome] was a scene to remember—a moment of theatrical drama; a moment so unusual in modern world athletics, when a virtual unknown from an insignificant country crosses the seas and conquers the heroes. It is a fine, unsophisticated, illogical victory."

How did winning a 26.2-mile race by outdueling the world's fastest marathoners end up being interpreted as an "illogical victory?"

In fact, Bikila had made a very rational decision to ditch the Adidas shoes since they might have given him painful blisters and possibly forced a withdrawal during the marathon. Furthermore, how were his racing tactics "unsophisticated"? He had held back for the first half the race, saving his energy for the second half. It was a brilliant, barefoot performance.

Nor was there anything "unsophisticated and illogical" when four years later, Bikila, now sponsored by Puma and wearing its shoes, repeated his marathon win at the Tokyo Olympics by setting another world record of 2:12:11. Well, that victory was not entirely supported by logic. Thirty-six days before the Olympics, he had undergone an appendectomy, and stayed in shape by jogging on the hospital grounds.

At the 1968 Mexico Olympics, Bikila wasn't as fortunate, dropping out around the ten-mile mark due to a training-related injury in his right knee. Then a year later, life took a tragic turn for Ethiopia's beloved, athletic hero. A car accident left him permanently paralyzed from the waist down. He died shortly afterwards at the age of forty-one.

Abebe Bikila is still widely remembered and revered in Ethiopia and elsewhere, especially among runners. When Vibram came out with its FiveFingers barefoot-style toe gloves, the footwear company named one of its models "Bikila." Yet the notion of literally following in Bikila's footsteps by racing shoeless in a marathon, or even at lesser distances, is one pretty much universally ignored by pro runners. Top marathoners from East Africa, despite having barefoot childhoods, almost all have shoe sponsorships that can range anywhere from $10,000 to $100,000 per year. Why would they ever want to walk away from this income stream? Yet among recreational runners, especially here in the US, the mere mention of barefoot running inspires a heated debate that's divided into two camps: a passionate minority of pro-barefoot or minimalist-shoe believers, whose bible is *Born to Run*, and everyone else.

My opinion on this subject has been the same for over thirty-five years. I even wrote a book called *Fix Your Feet* that came out in 2003. I spend as much time as possible barefoot and have done so my entire life. The issue of whether running shoes help or hurt a runner is exceptionally complex. There is no room for blindly worshiping the running shoe, nor should we shun them as the evil that barefoot purists claim. Because it's the runner's bare feet that will lead him to a 1:59 marathon. Not the shoes. I believe that a healthy, highly trained runner, would have already clocked a 1:59 marathon had the large footwear companies not muscled their way into the sport by offering lucrative shoe deals to top pro distance runners, especially those from Kenya.

Many of these Kenyan runners, who grew up in rural areas, spent almost all of their youth not wearing shoes. As a result, they developed highly efficient natural gaits by running barefoot.

"Virtually every successful Kenyan runner is from a poor, rural family," writes Adharanand Finn, a British journalist and author of *Running with the Kenyans*. "From an early age they run everywhere. Daniel Komen, the world-record holder at 3,000 meters, told me: 'Every day I used to milk the cows, run to school, run home for lunch, back to school, home, tend the cows. This is the Kenyan way.'"

Even when Kenyan kids aren't making daily trips on foot to school, they continue to run. That's because they have a real love for the sport, nurtured in large part by the success it might offer later in life. Here's Finn again: "Up in the Rift Valley, every village has its star runner, someone who has gone off to win a world title or some big city marathon, and returned with enough money to buy a plot of land, a cow and a big car. There are role models everywhere. The children look around them and say, when I grow up, I want to be a runner."

These children often compete in local all-comers' races. Almost all show up barefoot. Winners usually receive a free pair of shoes as their first-prize award. The shoes could be Fila, Puma, Nike, or Adidas. These brands are clearly a status symbol in running meccas like Kenya's Rift Valley. Just owning a pair of athletic shoes can be a young Kenyan's first taste of a possible career as a pro runner.

UNDERSTANDING OUR FEET

The feet play a primary role in developing and maintaining an optimal gait, preventing injuries, and assuring good running economy. The feet also create extra energy for running.

The foot, directly and indirectly, influences muscles, joints, ligaments, tendons and their movements throughout the body. This is accomplished from the ground up. In fact, many running injuries in the knees, hips, low back and other areas are caused by poor foot function, even in those individuals who don't have symptoms of imbalances in their feet.

The feet also generate energy. Each foot's impact with the ground, assisted by muscles and tendons in the legs, provides potential power for forward propulsion. Optimal, fully developed "recoil energy" significantly improves running economy, so a 2:04 marathoner may already be within reach of 1:59.

To better understand foot function, let's briefly review the differences between how humans walk and how they run. The major contrast between walking and *proper* (midfoot and forefoot) running is how the foot muscles function. The legs of a walking body act more like an inverted pendulum, swinging along step-by-step and while the knees remain locked.

Things significantly change with running, whereby a unique mechanism called *elastic recoil* occurs. The runner's movements are in the form of a springy gait, rebounding along on compliant legs and unlocked knees. This natural gait actually produces another source of additional power—the leg and foot have a built-in "return energy" system. This involves the Achilles and other tendons that actually recycle the impact energy of each step. (This return-energy mechanism has nothing to do with specious claims made by footwear companies that their running shoes have an energy-return system built into the soles; they don't—it's simply marketing hype.)

During natural running, many of the foot muscles don't technically push you off the ground like what happens during walking. Instead, the muscles provide an isometric-type tension to stabilize the tendons and help in the recycling of elastic energy for propelling the body forward. The large springy Achilles tendon on the back of the heel that runs up the leg and attaches into the large calf muscles (the gastrocnemius and soleus) plays a key role in recycling energy for propulsion. This and other tendons must function with sufficient tension to help in the return-energy process, and the muscles they attach to require a certain level of tautness, even at rest.

Trying to "loosen" the muscles and tendons associated with the recoil mechanism through stretching, aggressive massage, or other therapy may be counter-productive, impairing the natural springy gait. An injury of the calf muscles (usually associated with weakness, such as a "pulled" muscle) can also disturb the gait. Likewise, *excessive* tightness of the muscles that control the Achilles can be problematic too—it's a question of balance.

Those with shorter, more compact Achilles tendons, unlike taller runners who have longer heel bones attached to the Achilles, generally have a more efficient spring mechanism and better running economy—one reason why shorter runners may be better suited to run 1:59. For example, the late Kenyan Samuel Wanjiru, who took gold in the marathon at the 2008 Beijing Olympics in a record time of 2:06:32, and then followed that victory with wins at the London Marathon and Chicago Marathon (twice), was just 5-foot-4.

When a runner's foot properly hits the ground, impact energy is first stored in the muscles and tendons. Right away, 95 percent of this energy is then used to help spring the body forward like a pogo stick. This mechanism provides about half the energy required for leg- and foot-muscle propulsion, with the other half coming from sugar and fat metabolism.

This return-energy process can be affected several ways, resulting in some or much of the impact energy dissipated and lost:

- By landing on heels instead of the mid- or forefoot
- By overstriding
- When wearing over-supported shoes, especially ones that don't precisely match the foot
- When muscle imbalance is present in the legs or feet

Impairment of the return-energy process requires the runner to make up for this deficit by contracting muscles which then use more fat and sugar for fuel. The result is that the gait worsens and running economy is reduced. What happens next is that the pace slows, and for elite marathoners this can add several minutes or more to the finish time.

Foot and leg muscles play a key role in this energy-return system. This is because tendons attach muscles to bones. As studies demonstrate, less flexible runners are *more* economical in their gaits than those who have greater flexibility. Of course, being too inflexible or excessively flexible increases the risk of injury. So the 1:59 marathoner should *not* stretch as part of his training routine, relying instead on a proper active warm-up to allow the body to obtain its optimal, natural level of flexibility. Simply put, additional stretching makes the tendons more flexible in the feet and calf, and this leads to less energy obtained from impact forces resulting in a worsening running economy.

Dr. Rachael Drew and her colleagues at Penn State Heart and Vascular Institute, College of Medicine, explain it as follows: "This negative relationship is likely due to increased storage and return of elastic energy in stiffer musculotendinous structures during the stretch-shortening cycle, which reduces the aerobic demand of submaximal running. Body-heat generation is also minimized by rapid and efficient reutilization of this stored energy. In other words, less flexible runners are more economical."

There is no doubt that modern feet have been severely damaged by wearing narrow, ill-fitting shoes. Dr. Daniel Lieberman, professor of human evolution at Harvard, has spent a lot of time both in the lab and in the field looking at the human fossil record and biomechanics of how humans run. His research has taken him to Kenya where he videotaped runners. The filming provided accurate analysis of gait and footstriking. He argues that "most experienced, habitually barefoot runners tend to avoid landing on the heel and instead land with a forefoot or midfoot strike. The bulk of our published research explores the collisional mechanics of different kinds of foot strikes. We show that most forefoot and some midfoot strikes (shod or barefoot) do not generate the sudden, large impact transients that occur when you heel strike (shod or barefoot) . . . consequently, runners who forefoot or midfoot strike do not need shoes with elevated cushioned heels to cope with these sudden, high transient forces that occur when you land on the ground." In other words, avoid heel striking, whether you wear flat shoes or are barefoot. (Flat shoes are closer to being barefoot, while those with thicker soles, especially in the heels, can create an improper gait.)

Lieberman also wrote that being barefoot is about 5 percent more efficient than wearing shoes. This improvement in running economy is huge. It is another reason that I think many existing elite marathoners have the potential of going 1:59.

East African runners have a significant advantage. As children and often into adulthood, their bodies physically matured without interference from shoes. The Kenyan or Ethiopian way—growing up without shoes that can impede the development of the body's delicate and important running mechanics—may be one of the most important and unique features of their population.

Western children are not so fortunate. This may explain why distance runners from countries such as Australia, New Zealand, England, and the US haven't been able keep up with the East Africans. From the earliest age, even before children can walk, shoes are encouraged as being absolutely necessary. This is sadly the case, despite scientific and medical evidence to the contrary. For several decades, medical journals have published the science behind how shoes can harm the young human body, and also help cause physical ailments that appear in adulthood. Pediatricians, orthopedists, and many other physicians and health professionals have campaigned against the use of stiff modern shoes for young children and adolescents.

Rather than allowing the foot to develop naturally, almost all "modern" shoes have narrow toe boxes that don't allow the feet to widen as they should. So the foot becomes physically altered, and this frequently leads to poor neuromuscular development. It gets worse. Most shoes have thick soles and outsized heels. The net effect is that the feet can't communicate properly with the brain. Sensory perception is lost due to shoes. The entire body is adversely affected, including the brain. These harmful shoes are often overpriced and backed by multi-million dollar ad campaigns aimed at both adults, who buy the shoes, and children who want them. Runners are equally subject to the misleading marketing hype of the major shoe companies.

CHOOSING A SHOE, OR NOT

It's important to spend a considerable amount of time being barefoot during one's early development. Once the body and brain finish developing, by around age eighteen to twenty, wearing shoes that fit very well and are flat so as not to impede foot function may be much less harmful. Afterwards, maintaining one's barefoot state can help preserve the benefits gained during physical and neurological development. This includes spending time training without shoes.

For example, the training runs of Herb Elliott, of Australia, who was the world-record holder in the mile (3:54.5) and took gold in the 1,500 meters in the same Rome Olympics that Bikila won the marathon, were often done barefoot on the beach. One of the world's best middle-distance runners in the late 1950s and early 1960s, Elliott trained under the watchful eye of legendary coach Percy Cerutty, who believed in an holistic approach to athleticism, from eating healthy to reading philosophical classics to being barefoot. This unconventional approach worked. From 1957 to 1961, Elliott (wearing track spikes in competition) never lost a 1,500-meter or one-mile race. When he appeared for the first time on the cover of *Sports Illustrated*, he was photographed running barefoot on the beach.

While Elliott never competed at the longer distance of the marathon, his successful career offers strong evidence that training barefoot can give an elite marathoner a better chance of getting to 1:59. Furthermore, the potential of reaching that new running threshold is likely enhanced by racing barefoot. Let's look at the reasons why:

- A healthy barefoot state can improve running economy.
- The all-important recoil energy-generating mechanism in the foot and leg may be more effective barefoot.
- The balance of a foot's ground time and airtime is best barefoot. This allows sufficient ground time to obtain recoil energy (but too much also slows the pace).
- Training barefoot, when properly done, could reduce the risk of injury by keeping muscles better balanced.
- The extra weight of shoes, even lightweight racing flats, can lead to slower times.

But how much time can be potentially lost by wearing shoes in a marathon? Three factors play a role here. First is how the runner has developed the body and brain, starting from infancy, and while ensuring that the purest, most natural environment for the feet—being barefoot—isn't disrupted. The more time spent barefoot the better.

Second is how the shoes affect a runner's gait, recoil mechanism and other factors associated with muscle balance, especially later in the race as fatigue become more relevant. Shoes that don't perfectly match each foot can cause muscle imbalance, significantly reducing economy and pace. While this has never been accurately measured in a laboratory (it's a difficult task), one thing is certain—a runner wearing the wrong shoes will disturb the gait and elastic-recoil mechanism. This includes, for example, shoes with thick heels or other built-up soles that force runners to land on their heels.

The third factor is the weight of the shoe. How much can this add to one's marathon time? The results of tests performed by track coach Dr. Jack Daniels many years ago when he worked for Nike sheds light on how dramatic this amount could be. He tested runners on a treadmill using various weights added to shoes. Now associate professor of physical education at A. T. Stills College in Mesa, Arizona, Daniels demonstrated that this could be a reduction in running economy of one percent. For a marathon runner, this could be about a minute or more added to the finishing time for every 3.5-ounces of shoe weight. Yet almost all running shoes are between five and ten ounces—in dry weight.

We still don't know with any precise accuracy what the time difference is between wearing shoes and running barefoot, because there are many factors to consider. One is that everyone is an individual, and the response to wearing a shoe varies considerably. Hypothetically, given two marathoners of the same ability, one wearing lightweight racing flats and the other barefoot, expect the shoeless runner to finish ahead.

While the lightweight upper material of a racing shoe sheds water easily, it can still get damp. During a race, this may come from fluids that a runner spills while drinking from a paper cup or pouring water over his head, as well as sweat absorbed from the skin of the feet and ankles. It only takes a couple of tablespoons of liquid to make up one ounce of weight, especially if wearing socks (whose dry weight may be an additional half ounce)—each extra ounce of weight can slow one's marathon time by twenty seconds or more.

GROUND TIME VS. AIRTIME

The running foot spends part of its time on the ground, and the other part in the air, a situation influenced significantly by shoes. The balance of ground time and airtime is important when it comes to improving economy.

The part of a runner's gait that causes the most slowing of pace is when the foot is on the ground. Too much ground time can occur in two situations. One is during heel striking, a common phenomenon by runners who wear over-protected shoes with thick soles and outsized heels. This even includes some of today's popular racing flats. Another factor is over-striding. While many age group runners do this, even elites fall into the trap of over-striding when fatigue sets in. In both situations, the foot stays on the ground longer, further slowing the pace. When wearing shoes, the additional ground time is also due to the added weight and reduced muscle control.

But with great biomechanics, airtime and ground time are balanced, with the foot's contact with the ground providing a significant source of energy to move forward more economically, but without excess time to slow the pace. Two factors can help achieve this balance: cadence and the "hot-coal" technique.

CADENCE AND HOT COALS

Most of us run about 180 steps per minute. (We walk at a basic pace of about 120 steps per minute, a rate seen even when performing our daily activities.) An exception to the 180 number occurs when the feet adversely alter the body's gait, reducing the ability to maintain a healthy tempo. The result is that the body slows down. (Another exception is running on a treadmill, which is unnatural—the brain senses the body's movement but remains in one place. The result is a wider variation in tempo.)

The number 180 is not precise but an average. Virtually all runners have a range of tempo between about 150 and 190 steps a minute whether jogging, running a marathon, or sprinting. This allows the brain some leeway to adjust one's pace as necessary. Muscle fatigue, caffeine, time of day, the weather, and other factors can influence the cadence. In a race, the brain will sense these and other factors to make appropriate changes, such as slightly slowing one's tempo, or speeding it up, and increasing or decreasing stride length.

For decades, I've used the "hot-coal technique" to successfully help runners keep their feet off the ground as much as possible yet still rely on impact energy for added speed. Here's how it works: if you were running on hot coals, the moment your foot hit the hot surface you would want to raise it quickly. During any run, at the moment of impact the brain should already be telling foot, leg, thigh, pelvis, trunk and other muscles to begin contracting to lift the foot up off the ground. Performing this simple technique can help minimize ground time. It's much more practical when wearing flat-soled shoes, and easiest and most natural when barefoot. Think about this next time you run, and you'll easily be able to keep your foot from too much ground time while obtaining the benefits of return energy. When properly done, it will lower the heart rate at the same pace, or increase the pace at the same heart rate.

BAREFOOT THERAPY

How can the Kenyans, Ethiopians, or other elite runners, who are dependent on income from shoe sponsorships, improve their own foot function? Whether one grew up barefoot or not, the issue is how can a runner fix his feet and correct the damage incurred by wearing harmful shoes. Fortunately, it's cheap to correct feet. There is no huge expense or costly treatment when it comes to their rehabilitation—and it's something all runners can do, whether one is a recreational marathoner or a sub 2:10 pro.

Since the mid-1970s, running shoes started having thicker soles, more rigid support, and extra cushioning. Many people were running for the first time, and the shoe companies addressed this huge consumer demand by coming out with new models each year. (It was as if they were taking their lead from car companies.) Almost all running shoes used to be lightweight, flat, and flexible. Then as running became more popular, and large numbers of runners began getting injured from poor training or faulty biomechanics, footwear companies felt that shoes needed to have even more support and cushioning. Over the past thirty years, shoes continued getting beefier and bulkier. In time, the modern running shoe looked quite different than what was commonly available in the late 1960s and early 1970s.

But this development has not been kind to either the foot or the runner's gait.

When I give lectures to running clubs or groups of athletes, I often make a simple demonstration. First, I would ask a person who is wearing a popular running shoe (thick soles and outsized heels) to run across the stage in full view of the audience. Then I'd ask the subject to remove his or her shoes and run again, only this time barefoot. The difference would often be night-and-day. Instead of landing on the heels, going barefoot meant striking more mid- and forefoot. As a result, the entire body moves forward with a better, more balanced gait. The barefoot demo was usually sufficient to convince audience members to rethink their own footwear choices.

Getting rid of your thick-soled, over-supported shoes can be a big change for your feet. Spending more time barefoot can help this transition go smoother. Even when properly transitioning out of bad shoes, runners are still left with damaged feet. This typically includes muscle imbalances as a primary impairment. Correcting the problem is the goal of barefoot therapy. While some runners can breeze through the therapeutic steps outlined below, others will take longer. The differences include how long one has worn improper shoes as an adult, and how much barefoot time was spent as a child. Either way, the results can be dramatic.

10 Barefoot Steps

Here then are 10 barefoot steps that can lead to a better gait, and improve running economy. These steps are equally applicable to a 2:10 or 4:10 marathoner.

1. Take off your shoes. Don't put them on in the morning, unless you're going right outdoors. When coming home, take them off before walking into your house or apartment. Spend more time standing, walking and otherwise being barefoot. It's best without socks, but a good-fitting, thin pair is acceptable. Walk on the bare floor, carpeted areas, and wherever your feet take you. This provides different types of foot stimulation to help muscles work better—the first step in rehabilitating your feet. Do this for a week or two before moving onto the next step.

2. Now, take the plunge and venture outdoors in your bare feet. This will provide additional foot stimulation. Stick with smooth surfaces at first—a driveway, sidewalk, or porch. Do

this for at least ten minutes. The different environment—the feel of new materials by your bare feet, including temperature changes—provides added foot stimulation. A week or so of this additional activity and you're ready for the next stage.

3. Now try uneven natural ground. Walking on grass, dirt, and sand will provide greater motivation for your feet to function better. Start with just a few minutes if your feet feel sensitive, but with three weeks of barefoot training, you'll be ready for the following big step: working your way up to short walks of about ten to fifteen minutes.

4. During this rehab period, there are two important things to do with your shoes. First, start wearing thinner, simple footwear without supports. And second, make sure all the shoes you slip your feet into are a perfect fit.

5. Almost all runners can take these first four steps. It will help improve the body's mechanics from toe to head. But many people need further foot stimulus for additional rehabilitation. Being barefoot will do this eventually, but you can speed the process. Here's one effective way: foot massage. A professional massage is always wonderful to receive, but you can treat your own feet daily at home, either by yourself or trading treatments with others. Even a five-minute massage for each foot can work wonders. Start with the feet relaxed, clean, and dry. A small amount of organic coconut oil is a nice option. Slowly and gently rub the foot all over using both hands, working up the leg where key foot muscles originate. Use firm pressure, but it should not be painful. Do this daily or as often as possible.

6. A key feature of optimal foot function is overall body balance. Wearing shoes can significantly diminish this balance. Being

barefoot more often will help, but here is another way to get there faster. You should be able to easily balance on one bare foot for thirty seconds or more. If you can't perform this action, it's probably due to foot dysfunction. Start with attempting to balance on one foot for as long as you can, even if just for a few seconds; next, try the other foot. Balancing on each foot can gradually improve the communication between feet and brain, thereby promoting better balance throughout the body. Try to incorporate this therapeutic activity into a regular routine: After a shower or bath—hold one foot up to dry and massage it while standing on the other. Be sure to get each of your toes, and keep your foot relaxed. Then switch feet. Here's another good routine: each day when putting on your shoes, do it standing, holding your foot above your knee to put on the shoe and tie it, then do the same with the other.

7. By the end of the day, many runners have tired, sore, and hot feet. The solution: cool them down. A cold footbath can work wonders, even after a hot shower. It helps circulation, tones muscles, and improves foot function. Use a large enough bucket or foot tub that fits your feet without jamming the toes. Place your feet in cold water so they are completely submerged above the ankle. Add a small amount of ice to prevent the water from getting warm, but do not fill the tub with ice as this can freeze the foot, risking damage to nerves, blood vessels, and muscles. Keep your foot immersed for five to twenty minutes. A deeper bath can also cool the leg muscles. A cold footbath can do much more than an ice pack placed only on an area of discomfort. Take a footbath

while answering email, catching up on phone calls, or use it as a time to relax and listen to music.

8. Sometimes, the use of a hot footbath can be therapeutic, not to mention comforting. Moist heat works better than a heating pad because it penetrates into the foot better. Use the same size footbath as mentioned above, and fill with hot water—not scalding—but most people can tolerate temperatures of around 95-100 degrees Fahrenheit. Adding Epsom salt (magnesium salt) is also soothing. Beware: heat comes with contraindications. Do not use heat if you have an acute injury, especially one that's inflamed, swollen, or bruised, and avoid heat with any skin disorder, diabetes, circulatory problem, or an open wound. When in doubt about using heat, avoid it.

9. By now it may be time to turn your outdoor barefoot experience into an easy jog or run. There are many ways to describe this process, but like other natural activities, your body already knows how to do it. Begin on blacktop, or smooth dirt, since this will allow the body to adapt by naturally thickening the skin on the bottoms of the feet. Ultimately, you may be able to run anywhere barefoot. Use this barefoot time as a warm-up for your longer run in flat shoes, a cool down, or maintain it as a separate therapy. Many athletes take this as a launching pad for regular barefoot running, whether it's a 45-minute workout or even running in races.

10. This final step is critical. Once you have weaned yourself from harmful shoes, rehabbed your feet, and restored good foot function, be careful to avoid returning to old unhealthy habits by wearing bad shoes. It's that simple.

Finding the Perfect Fit

Finding a shoe that properly fits each of your feet should be a top priority. This will help you run longer distances on any terrain with less stress on the body. But the search for a great pair of shoes is easier said than done.

Always plan on spending adequate time when shopping for shoes. Don't rush—if you're short on time, postpone it and set time aside for this important event. You may not find the right shoes in the first store you visit. Most outlets carry only a few of the many shoes on the marketplace.

You can get the best fit by following some key points:

- Use comfort as the primary factor in finding the best fit. Don't let the store employee or manager say that you have to "break them in" before they feel good. The best shoes feel good right away. (Shoes from mail-order outlets may cost less, but be prepared to ship them back if they don't fit just right.)
- Never assume you'll take the same size as your previous shoe, even if it's the same type or model. The shoe industry does not have standardization when it comes to sizes—company A's size 10 shoes are a bit larger than company B's size 10.
- Because each foot is different, always try on both shoes. As a general guide, try the size you think would fit best then walk on a hard floor (not carpeted). Even if that size feels fine, try on a half-size larger. If that one feels the same, or even better, try on another half-size larger. Many people don't realize that a larger shoe may actually feel and fit better.

- Continue trying on larger half-sizes until you find the shoes that are obviously too large. You will know especially by the heel—it will start lifting off when you walk. Then go back to the previous half-size—more often that's the pair that best matches your feet. There should be at least a half-inch between your longest toe and the front of the shoe for most shoes.
- Each time you try on a pair of shoes, find a hard surface to walk on rather than the thick soft carpet in shoe stores, where almost any shoe will feel good. If there's no sturdy floor to walk on, ask if you can walk outside (if you're not allowed, shop elsewhere).
- You may also need to try different widths to get the best fit, although many shoes don't come in different widths. The ball of your foot should fit comfortably into the widest part of the shoe without causing the shoe to bulge.
- If the difference between your two feet is less than a half-size, fit the larger foot. If you have a significant difference of more than a half-size between your two feet, it may be best to wear two different-size shoes. How you accomplish this is up to you.
- With what you think is the best-fitting shoe, run on a hard surface. They should still fit great with continued, almost perfect comfort.

The odds of a 1:59 marathon are stacked in favor of a shoeless runner. When we examine the human foot and its relationship to gait and biomechanics, the running shoe just might be the final barrier blocking an elite marathoner from accomplishing this historic feat. And just because the top marathoners, many of whom grew up running barefoot, choose to professionally compete in shoes, this doesn't mean that they can't return to their shoeless roots. It might take some time for these runners to make that transition and go back to being barefoot. But they should remember that when all their running as youth was done barefoot, it was how they developed their natural, fluid gaits.

Top runners will wear those shoes that make them run the fastest. In fact, many elite runners wear shoes made by companies other than the ones given them by their sponsor. They secretly do this because the quest for the ideal racing shoe is nearly an obsession, as it should be considering how footwear affects the whole body.

Let's take this discussion even one step further—once a contemporary shoeless runner wins a big-city marathon (such as Boston, New York City, London, Berlin, or Tokyo), other pro and elite runners will follow his example. Don't be surprised if the first marathoner to go 1:59 is barefoot. That runner could be a Kenyan, Ethiopian, or a runner from another country. Our barefoot 1:59 marathoner will change the sport of running overnight. It will also disrupt the footwear industry in many positive ways.

CHAPTER 10

NUTRITION

You Are What You Eat

> — Title of best-selling book in 1940 by nutritionist DR. VICTOR
> LINDLAHR, an early pioneer and advocate of healthy food

Travel to a country like Kenya and Ethiopia, and you expect to find most of the population on the lean side, unlike what you see in the industrialized West where obesity is a major problem. But this is changing. The East African nations are in the midst of what the World Health Organization (WHO) calls the *nutrition transition.* The diet shift is also occurring in almost all developing countries in the Third World. In just a single generation, obesity rates have skyrocketed, with sedentary youth most at risk. This health crisis is particularly apparent in cities, where refined carbohydrates, soft drinks, and cheap junk food are easily accessible.

The scenario in rural areas where the population is more active is much different. Go to a small village in Kenya's Rift Valley, and here the barefoot youth seem always in motion, running to school and doing farm work. Being overfat is not a health issue. At least, so far.

The elite runners who live and train here are thin and sinewy. They don't follow a special diet tailored to endurance. Nor do they load up on sports drinks, energy bars, or mineral supplements. They eat the same foods that everyone in their village also eats.

The most popular dishes in Kenya are *ugali* (a bland corn mush), *githeri* (a mixture of boiled corn and kidney beans), and *sukuma wiki* (chopped boiled kale). Meat is in short supply, so many runners eat it sparingly. A common snack for these endurance athletes is roasted corn on the cob without salt. They also love their tea, heavily doused with sugar.

The bodies of Kenyan runners are in constant need of energy replenishment due to all the training; they eat for fuel and not necessarily for taste. "They eat food eaten by ordinary Kenyans," a senior lecturer at Kenyatta University's Department of Exercise Science recently told National Public Radio in 2012. "The cook is not a sports dietician, just a woman from the village."

Should all runners follow the Kenyan diet? Many curious, elite marathoners in the Western world probably have already sampled their bland, packed-with-calories fare. (Just as many runners in the US took a sudden interest in "energy-boosting" chia seeds and pinole, a staple of the Tarahumara Indians, after reading *Born to Run*.) If this small nation that's comprised of forty-two ethnic tribes—most pro runners are Kalenjin, which has a population of 2.5 million or 11 percent of Kenya's total—can produce the fastest distance runners, then doesn't it logically follow that its endurance athletes must be eating right? The answer, surprisingly, is a definite no. But there is even a more relevant question: *How much faster could the Kenyans run if they stuck to a healthier diet?*

The Kenyan diet is lacking; it's nutritionally substandard. Total daily protein amounts, along with a variety of vitamins and minerals are low even by the modest Recommended Daily Allowance (RDA) standards. There's also an excess quantity of refined carbohydrate and processed fats. In 2004, a nutritional study published in the *International Journal of Sport Nutrition and Exercise Metabolism* examined the diets of several elite Kenyan runners. The study found most of their nutrients were from vegetable sources, with the main items being bread, boiled rice, poached potatoes, boiled porridge, cabbage, kidney beans, and *ugali*. A whopping 76 percent of their daily calories came from carbohydrates, mostly refined. Meat was consumed, but only in small portions, averaging four times a week (3.5-ounce servings).

The Kenyan runners' chronically deficient diet can lead to health problems that often begin by their early twenties and worsen in their thirties, with an increase of injuries and illnesses in what should be their prime. There's also a subtle increase in body fat.

The effects of poor, long-term nutrition among East African runners should be a wake-up call if they want to remain on top.

A review of the top fifty fastest marathon times indicates that most of these runners are either apparently past their peak or too frequently injured to maintain their stellar racing performances. Geoffrey Mutai and Wilson Kipsang may be the only solid exceptions—both in their early thirties and candidates for a 1:59, and they each have a long string of strong performances between 2009 and 2013. Ethiopian Haile Gebrselassie, one of the all-time greatest distance runners, had an amazing career, but it might have prematurely ended due to asthma and other preventable health issues.

What does the future hold for the next generation of East African runners? As scientists point out, poor nutrition early in life adversely affects metabolism, which can increase the risks of ill health in adulthood. Though most of the top East African runners grew up in poor in a rural environment, life in the country is changing, with eating habits becoming more like those found in the cities, including the consumption of refined carbohydrates such as white flour, processed food, and soft drinks.

When Kenyan and Ethiopian runners come to Europe and the US in order to race, they are further exposed to the West's junk-food lifestyle, with Starbucks, Pizza Hut, and McDonald's on almost every corner in the large cities. All of this makes for a potentially debilitating scenario for today's young, up-and-coming East African runners. By the time they hit their thirties, and perhaps not winning or placing high as often, the health damage might already be too permanent to reverse.

Will bad diets mark the beginning of the end for East African dominance in distance running? It's hard to know with any certainty, especially because the region has a nearly bottomless pool of running talent from which it annually draws upon. But as the junk-food diet continues to migrate from Nairobi to the countryside, Kenya's young, talented runners might not be able to escape its harmful effect on overall health.

The situation is so much worse in this country. When it comes to the manufacture and consumption of unhealthy food, the US leads the world. Even our most fit, active athletes are affected. Many of America's top distance runners follow a similar ritual when it comes to diet. It goes like this: wolf down pancakes, cereal, or a bagel for breakfast, a big lunch containing plenty of pasta and bread, snacks through the day of so-called energy bars or sports drinks packed with carbs, and dinner might include fish or meat, along with more processed-food side dishes and a sugary dessert or two.

This type of diet is counter-productive if one wants to improve as a runner. And it's more than simply carbo-loading nearly every day of the week. These foods actually undermine one's training because they are just a lot of sugar in various forms, void of real nutrition, and typically increase body fat.

The subject of diet and nutrition is quite vast. I have written hundreds of articles and close to a dozen books that extensively cover this topic. So what are the best foods for runners? To answer this question, there are two effective approaches. One is to highlight each important macronutrient (carbohydrate, fat and protein), micronutrient (the 40-plus vitamins and minerals), phytonutrient (some 25,000 of them), and other items such as calories. The other is to emphasize the consumption of real, healthy foods, which already contains these nutrients. I will use the latter approach here.

Let's start with the basics. Healthy foods form the foundation of a successful running program because they directly and indirectly help the body in the following ways:

- Generate maximum amounts of energy from fat for aerobic speed
- Correct and prevent muscle imbalance and other injuries
- Encourage optimal brain function
- Promote faster recovery from training and racing
- Maintain high-quality blood cells to carry oxygen to muscles
- Prepares one for optimal performance on race day

Healthy food is critical for runners. Each day the body breaks down during the catabolic phase of training. With the anabolic phase of recovery the body is rebuilt, repaired, and made stronger. The raw materials necessary for this revitalization come from the foods we eat. The best foods create a superior body—simply put, we are what we eat.

REAL FOOD VS. JUNK FOOD

When it comes to food selection, there are really just two choices. Real food provides the necessities to build the best runner. Junk food does not, and is harmful.

- *Real food* is naturally occurring, unadulterated and unprocessed, and nutrient-rich. If you can grow or raise food, it's real. Included are fresh fruits and vegetables, lentils and beans, eggs, real cheese, whole pieces of meat (such as fish, beef, chicken), nuts, seeds, and similar items. Consuming these foods provide a great potential for both immediate and long-term health benefits. This is the foundation of sports nutrition, not only for daily meals and snacks, but also for pre- and post-race needs.

- *Junk food* is everything else. It's deceptively inexpensive and easy to buy, and unhealthy to eat. These items include processed, manufactured foods with added chemicals, sugars and other unhealthy ingredients that can immediately, and long term, adversely affect health and performance. Canned fruit in sugar-syrup, processed vegetables (also canned, frozen, or from fast food outlets) with sugar, various types of refined flour and instant foods, baked beans in a sugar and flour sauce, powdered and processed eggs with trans fats, fake cheese spreads, cold cuts (bologna, salami, chicken and turkey loaf, fish sticks), peanut butter (typically containing sugar and trans fat), and roasted nuts (often with ingredients that are difficult to pronounce) are some examples. Of course, genetically altered items, which are not allowed in certified organic foods or in many countries of the world, would also be considered junk food, as are most sports products, including so-called energy bars, drinks, and powders.

And as most people know, junk food, especially sugar and white flour, is a primary cause of the worldwide overfat epidemic that's affecting the full spectrum of individuals, from the poor to the most serious athletes. In addition to increasing body fat, junk food—and that includes anything that contains processed white flour or added sugar—may be the number-one cause of the most common diseases, including cancer, diabetes, Alzheimer's, and heart disease, not to mention the problems that significantly contribute to low quality of life such as intestinal conditions, hormone imbalance, chronic inflammation, fatigue, and much more. These conditions are also found among many runners. Fitness is little guarantee of being healthy if one's diet is unsound.

Some health and diet authorities want to refer to junk food as *pathogenic* food. But that won't happen soon enough thanks to the ongoing multi-million-dollar marketing campaigns waged by the food and beverage industry—these bad foods and drinks are portrayed as harmless rather than the poison they really are. Even most health food stores carry junk food—some of it is in the form of packaged organic items.

Junk foods and drinks have been promoted as a necessary part of sports nutrition for many years. It's another scam by companies selling these products, masked as something endurance athletes sorely need. Junk food is also one of the world's most successful business ventures. Not surprisingly, even Kenya now has fast food restaurants, including KFC and Subway. Along with Coke and other junk foods infiltrating East Africa, the criticism that these products are further contributing to obesity and disease are overshadowed by corporate profits.

REFINED CARBOHYDRATES

The most common junk-food ingredients are refined carbohydrates. They are also the worst food for marathoners. Refined carbs come in two forms, sugar and flour. There are many different versions of these basic junk-food ingredients.

Sugar comes in various identities including all maltose products (maltodextrin, malt sugar, maple sugar, and syrup), corn sugars and syrups (such as high-fructose corn syrup), all cane sugars (whether white, brown, or raw), rice syrups, and molasses. Many of these harmful ingredients are found in most energy bars and sports drinks. They should be avoided in a healthy diet.

When using sweeteners, the best one is a simple, natural carbohydrate called honey.

After they are consumed, most carbohydrates are broken down into its two simple sugars, glucose and fructose, then absorbed by the intestines into the blood. This immediately triggers the release of the hormone insulin from the pancreas. While insulin is a very important hormone, too much can be produced after eating refined carbohydrates; it then adversely affects one's endurance by reducing the ability to burn body fat.

After consuming carbohydrates, the body's insulin performs these important actions:

1. It helps convert about half the carbohydrates eaten into energy, especially for muscles and the brain.
2. Up to about 10 percent of the carbohydrates you eat are converted to glycogen, a storage form of sugar. This amount varies with how much is needed in the muscles and liver. (Muscle glycogen is

converted to glucose for energy, and liver glycogen helps maintain blood sugar levels between meals and during nighttime sleep.)

3. About 40 to 50 percent of the carbohydrates consumed are immediately converted to fat and stored in the body. While this is the fat used by the aerobic muscles for energy, if the fat-burning mechanism is not working well, or if too many carbohydrates are consumed, fat stores can increase.

Insulin is produced whenever carbohydrates are consumed. High amounts of refined carbohydrates, such as sugar and white flour, can impair the aerobic system by reducing the body's ability to burn fat for energy. This affects training and racing because of reduced aerobic speed. In fact, even a modest pre-treadmill test meal of cereal, pancakes, pasta, or an energy bar, can result in poor performance when measuring fat- and sugar-burning.

The exception to insulin production is when carbohydrates are consumed *during* training or competition; lower insulin levels help the body burn more stored fat for energy. (Insulin can also be produced with a high-protein meal as some amino acids convert to glucose.)

It's simple: the more refined carbohydrates consumed, the more insulin produced by the pancreas.

In addition to causing even more carbohydrates to convert and store as fat, excess insulin can continue lowering the blood sugar. Since the brain exclusively relies on glucose for fuel, periods of reduced blood sugar can result in decreased mental function, including reduced concentration—many athletes get sleepy after a meal too high in carbs. Low blood sugar also triggers hunger, sometimes only an hour or two after the meal. Cravings for sweets are typically part of this cycle and resorting to snacking on more carbohydrates seems nonstop. If you don't eat, you just feel worse.

This problem may appear relatively minor in younger runners because symptoms are often missing. But on the other extreme, especially in athletes who are approaching age thirty, there can be the following developments: higher body fat, elevations in blood pressure, or even diabetes. The full spectrum of this carbohydrate problem is a health condition that I long ago named as *carbohydrate intolerance*. It's the inability to cope with refined-carbohydrate intake.

The problem of refined-carbohydrate intake leading to elevated insulin can also suppress two important hormones: glucagon and growth hormone. Both are important for athletes. Glucagon promotes the use of both fat and sugar for energy. Growth hormone helps provide many benefits that one obtains through proper training, including muscle development, energy production, and the regulation of minerals and amino acids.

Rising insulin can also increase the stress hormone cortisol, which can lower another important hormone for athletes, and that is testosterone.

GLYCEMIC INDEX

The general measure of an increase in blood sugar after eating specific carbohydrates, and the associated rise in insulin, is referred to as the glycemic index (GI). High-GI foods, which trigger the most insulin, include cereal, bagels, breads, potatoes, sweets, and other foods that contain refined flour and sugar. Even foods that you may think are good for you can trigger high amounts of insulin, including fruit juice, maple syrup, and large bananas (especially when green/ unripe). Most sports drinks, energy bars, and other carbohydrate-based products are also very high on the glycemic index; they should only be used *during* training or competition when insulin levels are much lower, but not as a regular part of an athlete's diet.

Here are some examples of higher and lower glycemic foods:

Higher-Glycemic Foods
Refined flour products: bread, chips, bagels, cereals
Sugar and sugar-containing foods: candy, cookies, soda
Sweet fruits: pineapple, watermelon, grapes, bananas, all fruit juice
Starchy vegetables: potatoes, corn
Sports drinks and bars when used for meals or snacks

Lower-Glycemic Foods
Unrefined grains: whole rye and wheat kernels, wheat germ, quinoa
Lower-sugar fruits: apples, peaches, pears, berries, melons
Lentils, beans
All other vegetables

The use of carbohydrates during a marathon certainly has value. However, the primary focus of race energy is to first develop the aerobic system to generate additional energy from burning more body fat. With high levels of fat for energy, well-trained runners can easily perform a two-plus hour run at maximum aerobic heart rate without the need for further carbohydrates. Supplemental nutrients during a race is reduced or eliminated, since energy reserves from one's body fat are extensive. Only with a well-developed aerobic system already in place can one consider the merits of race nutrition.

RACE NUTRITION

Simple carbohydrates can play an essential role in race nutrition. Specifically, consuming carbohydrates during a marathon can help maintain higher levels of fat burning. This has to do with the body's complex metabolism, and the reliance of both sugar and fat for race energy.

Unfortunately, most sports products contain *complex* carbohydrates, which must be digested before the sugar is made available to help fat burning. Digestion is poor while running. The result is that many athletes consuming these products feel bloated or experience intestinal discomfort during a race.

The two best carbohydrates for racing are fruit juice and honey. But this needs to be emphasized: the issue of needing a carbohydrate drink during a marathon should be pre-determined during long training runs. Don't try something new on race day.

The two most important factors when using a carbohydrate beverage are the strength of the solution, and the type of sugar it contains.

The Carbohydrate Solution

The concentration or strength of the carbohydrate solution refers to the amount of sugar and water in the drink. Whether homemade or one of the many retail products available, the concentration can influence how your intestines tolerate the drink. Homemade liquid carbohydrate drinks are best because they are simple to make, are made from basic natural foods, don't contain unwanted or unhealthy ingredients (some are not listed on the label), and you can adjust the amount of carbohydrate for your particular needs. Unfortunately, obtaining these drinks during a race is not nearly as easy as making it.

A 6 to 8 percent carbohydrate solution is ideal for most marathoners during a race (and for longer training, if necessary). This can be made by adding six to eight grams of carbohydrate (approximately one heaping teaspoon), such as honey, to 90 ml (three ounces) of water.

This solution will not remain in your stomach very long but will empty into the small intestines at a similar rate as water. Liquids that are concentrated with more than 8 percent carbohydrate can remain in the stomach longer, not allowing the stomach to empty as fast, delaying the absorption of sugar, and often causing stomach to feel bloated or become upset.

My suggestion is to experiment. Always start by using liquids made of simple, natural sugars such as honey, or fruit juice, with apple working well and citrus being too acidic for most athletes. The sugar content of most commercial juices is 6 to 8 percent (not the concentrated versions, which are much higher).

Experiment during training, not racing. Find out which types of carbohydrate solutions make you feel the best, especially in your gut after consuming, and which seem to give you more energy and better recovery. Obviously, you will quickly learn to avoid those solutions that cause intestinal distress.

NO WATER STOP FOR 1:59

Our 1:59 marathoner probably won't need to consume any water or carbohydrate drink during his record-setting run. With that said, race conditions will influence his hydration status. On a dry, hot sunny day, a runner will lose more water through sweat, and dehydration may become excessive requiring some water intake. When cool and overcast, however, hydration is less problematic and consuming water may be unnecessary.

A healthy body regulates water extremely well. In a fast marathon, dehydration of about two to three percent may normally occur. This won't affect performance; in fact, it can actually help it.

This slight level of dehydration results in a significant reduction in body weight, especially later in the race. In a 140-pound runner, for example, this can equate to three to four pounds of a loss in water weight. (Recall that the weight of running shoes may be between five and ten ounces, and this slight extra weight had the potential of reducing an elite's marathon time by a minute.) While it's not possible to accurately estimate water weight loss in any one individual at various points along the race, it can obviously be a factor.

Hormones also play a key role in water regulation. In particular, the brain's hypothalamus and pituitary gland helps maintain balanced hydration by informing the kidneys to conserve or excrete water depending on conditions. Too much water loss during a race can cause serious dehydration and reduce performance. But drinking excessively can be a problem too, especially in the presence of hormone imbalance. It can lead to *water toxicity*, which can negatively impact both performance and health.

Closely associated with water regulation is a key electrolyte, sodium. Hormone imbalance in the adrenal glands can result in too much sodium loss leading to *hyponatremia* (low-blood sodium). Combined with excess water consumption, these two problems significantly impair performance, and could be life-threatening.

CREATE YOUR OWN ENERGY BARS AND POWER SHAKES

My favorite snack food is my own homemade energy bar. I call it Phil's Bar, though you won't find it in any health food store. It's a complete meal of low-glycemic carbohydrates with healthy protein and good fats—and easy to digest. And it tastes great. Here's the recipe:

3 cups whole almonds

⅔ cup powdered egg white

4 tablespoons pure powdered cocoa

½ cup unsweetened shredded coconut

Pinch of sea salt

⅓ cup honey

⅓ cup hot water

1 to 2 teaspoons vanilla

Grind dry ingredients in a food processor. Mix honey, hot water and vanilla together, and blend into dry ingredients. (At this point, you may have to mix it all by hand depending on your food processor). Shape into bars, cookies, or lightly press into a buttered muffin tin. You can also press the batter into a dish (about one-inch deep) and cut into squares. Adjust the water/honey ratio for less or more sweetness. Keep refrigerated (they'll still last a week or more out of the refrigerator). For other flavor options, use fresh lemon instead of cocoa, or use more coconut. Makes ten to twelve bars.

My favorite morning meal is a healthy shake (or smoothie). I also have one mid-afternoon. It's made with fresh, raw organic fruits and vegetables, raw seeds and fresh eggs for protein. One could use other protein sources such as fresh or powdered whey or egg whites. (I lightly soft-boil a dozen eggs at a time and keep them refrigerated, so preparation for this shake is about five minutes.)

Here's my large one-serving smoothie recipe:

1 large or 2 small apples, pears, peaches, or the best in-season fruits

2 soft cooked eggs

1 whole carrot

Spinach, kale, parsley, cilantro, beet root and/or greens (one to two servings)

About ½ cup blueberries

1 teaspoon plain psyllium (optional)

1 tablespoon coconut oil

1 tablespoon raw whole sesame and or flax seeds

8–10 ounces water

Add all ingredients to a good blender and mix well.

The best blenders will do a great job on the whole fruits, including the core and all the seeds, and the raw whole carrot, raw spinach, kale, cilantro, or other vegetables. With enough fruit for sweetness, none of the bitter taste from the vegetables is noticeable—you'd never know there were so many healthy ingredients!

Breaking the tradition of consuming large volumes of refined carbohydrates is an important step to reducing excess body fat, developing a more efficient aerobic system, and building a healthier body and brain. How many carbs should a runner consume? This, of course, depends on the individual. But a diet that is about a third carbohydrate—containing only natural sources—is more than adequate for most runners.

PROTEIN

While most of the great marathoners appear lean without much excess muscle, it is deceiving. A full 40 percent of one's body weight may be muscle (a bit less in females). Running requires the use of more body-wide muscles than virtually all other sports. Training results in a daily turnover of muscle that needs repair and replacement, which can be significant. How much dietary protein does this require? It varies with the individual. But because body weight is related to one's muscle mass, the following can be used as a guide.

Minimum daily protein needs may be about 1.6 grams of protein per kilogram of body weight, or about 0.7 grams per pound. Let's look at two examples:

- For a 145-pound runner, the requirement may be about 104 grams. This can be obtained from three eggs for breakfast, a large salmon filet for lunch, a medium sirloin steak for dinner, and two snacks of nuts, cheese, or other protein sources.
- A runner weighing 125 pounds would minimally require about 90 grams of protein. This can be obtained from two eggs at breakfast, a medium filet of fish for lunch, a lamb chop for dinner, and one snack of nuts, cheese, or other protein sources.

You can adjust the exact proportion to your own weight. By sticking to these guidelines, a runner will learn that a diet comprised of 30 percent protein might be about right.

The popular (and misunderstood) dietary trend in recent years has been against eating meat, but there are a variety of unique health features of animal foods that are vital for marathon training and racing. Here are some of them:

- Animal foods contain high levels of all amino acids.
- Vitamin B_{12} is an essential nutrient found only in animal foods.
- EPA, an essential fat that helps control inflammation, is almost exclusively found in animal foods.
- Iron is necessary for red blood cells to carry oxygen to muscles. Animal foods contain this mineral in the most bio-available form.

- Vitamin A is found only in animal products. Plant foods— including vegetables and fruits—contain only beta-carotene, which is not vitamin A; its conversion in the body to vitamin A is not always efficient in humans.

- Those who consume less animal protein have greater rates of bone loss than those who eat larger amounts of animal protein.

- The amino acid glutamine, the main energy source for optimal intestinal function, is primarily found in meat, especially those minimally cooked such as rare beef.

The best animal sources may be organic, grass-fed, free-range, kosher and whatever other labels are used to differentiate the highest quality eggs, meats, fish, and dairy foods from those obtained from poorly treated animals. Beware of the modern food-industrial complex, which mass produces beef, chicken, pork, and other animals in unhealthy (and often inhumane) ways. The result is dangerous food, typically found in the fast-food industry, with higher risks of *E. coli* outbreaks and items containing harmful hormones and chemicals used in the raising of animals and production of these foods.

The human intestinal track is well adapted for digesting animal-source foods, having evolved for several million years on a diet relatively high in meat and fish, with varying amounts of vegetables, fruits, and nuts.

OTHER NOTABLE NUTRIENTS

Research continues to demonstrate what nutrition-oriented clinicians and coaches have long known: certain foods help guide the body into overreaching and prevent the downward drifting into overtraining. These nutrients directly affect the rate of rest or recovery. They also help you avoid injury and illness, and will assist in improved muscle function. Two groups of nutrients found in the diet are vital for optimal training and racing—those associated with dietary fats that regulate inflammation, and antioxidants that control free radicals.

FATS AND INFLAMMATION

When a small cut breaks the skin of a finger, it swells, turns red and eventually heals. A similar process occurs after each training run—there's a breakdown of muscle and other tissues in the body, then they build back up. This recovery and repair process is governed to a great extent by inflammation. Let's look at the two forms of inflammation:

- Acute inflammation is a normal healthy action, helping to heal more than just that little cut on one's finger. The body relies on it as the first step in recovery from a workout so one can be ready for the next day's run. (A more extreme inflammatory response occurs after a marathon.)

Normally, the inflammatory mechanism acts like an "on-off" switch. The body's inflammatory chemicals are produced when recovery and repair are needed. Then the process is turned off by production of the body's anti-inflammatory chemicals. However, if the anti-inflammatory chemicals are not present in sufficient quantity, if the inflammatory chemicals are excessive, or there is an ongoing injury or stress (such as overtraining) that keeps stimulating inflammatory chemicals, the result can be *chronic inflammation*.

- Chronic inflammation is a common component of the overtraining syndrome, triggering those all-too-familiar "itis" conditions such as tendinitis, bursitis, and arthritis. In the long term, it is also a precursor to heart disease, cancer and other chronic illness.

Key nutrients in one's diet regulate inflammation. These are the *essential fats* called omega-6 and omega-3. When these fats are not balanced they can impair the body's ability to properly regulate inflammation. The most common problem for runners is that they consume too much omega-6 fat and too little omega-3.

Here are two important recommendations to balance these essential fats:

1. When using dietary fats and oils for cooking, use only butter or ghee ("drawn" or purified butter), coconut oil or lard.
2. Avoid all vegetable oil—soy, safflower, corn, canola and peanut—and trans fat (from margarine and other processed fats and oils). These are high in omega-6 oils and too much can impair the inflammatory process. Instead, use any of the above recommended cooking fats, or extra virgin olive oil.

The most important fat for runners is omega-3 which is best obtained in animal products because it contains the nutrient EPA (eicosapentaenoic acid). While fish is the optimal source, our oceans now have high levels of pollution, so it is optimal to rely on a dietary supplement of fish oil (in which the toxins have been removed). Vegetable sources of omega-3 fat such as flax and other seeds do not contain EPA (although the body converts a small amount of these oils to EPA, it is not adequate).

In addition to fats, certain foods can play a key role in helping to balance inflammation. These include ginger and turmeric, citrus peel (when eating the fruit, also consume some of the skin and white parts) and the onion family—shallots, chive, and garlic. *It should be noted that the consumption of sugar and refined flour (or any high-glycemic food) promotes excess inflammation even when fats are balanced.*

In a healthy diet containing good natural fats, which also include nuts and seeds, avocados, egg yolks, and fats from meats, about a third of a runner's total calories might come from fat.

ANTIOXIDANTS AND FREE RADICALS

Another vital part of the repair process that a runner undergoes each day is the production of chemicals called *free radicals*. We require a certain amount of these natural chemicals, but too much causes chronic inflammation, muscle fatigue, immune dysfunction and reduced training and racing performance. Free radicals may also be a primary factor contributing to overtraining. (Aerobic training does *not* produce an excess of free radicals, but anaerobic workouts and races do.)

The body controls free radicals with a large group of nutrients called *antioxidants*. There are probably thousands of antioxidants in a healthy diet, and scientists have yet to discover all of them. They include vitamins A, C and E, certain minerals such as selenium and zinc, and many phytonutrients that include bioflavanoids, carotenoids, phenols and many more. Most are found in fresh vegetables and fruits—the reason 10 servings of these foods each day is an important recommendation.

The most powerful antioxidant is one produced by the body. *Glutathione* is made from other dietary nutrients that include:

-   The amino acid cysteine found in animal protein, especially whey.

173

- Sulphoraphan is found in cruciferous vegetables such as broccoli, kale, and brussels sprouts. The highest content is in young, two- to three-day-old broccoli sprouts before their leaves turn green.

- Lipoic acid is found in many dark vegetables (spinach, broccoli, Brussels sprouts, whole peas) and grass-fed beef.

- Gamma-tocopherol and alpha-tocotrienol, parts of the vitamin E complex, are found in raw almonds and cashews, and sesame and flax seeds. (Beware: popular doses of alpha tocopherol—100 IU or more of vitamin E—can reduce some of the body's antioxidants.)

It's not necessary to remember the names of these antioxidants, but you do need to remember to eat as many antioxidant-rich foods as possible. These include a wide variety of vegetables and fruits, including blueberries and other berries, sesame seeds, almonds, extra virgin olive oil, green and black tea. Even red wine and beef are excellent sources of antioxidants.

Obtaining all of one's nutrition from healthy food should be a primary goal for all runners. In some situations, only then can the use of dietary supplements be considered as a means to obtain additional nutrients.

DIETARY SUPPLEMENTS

Many runners mistakenly believe that they must take daily dietary supplements. They might know that their diet is inadequate, so taking supplements should only help and not hurt. Right? But for many years a variety of studies have demonstrated the potential dangers of many types of supplements.

The fact that a dietary supplement contains nutrients does not mean it's natural, or even safe. In fact, the vitamins in almost all dietary supplements are synthetic. Most are made from artificial chemicals in a manufacturing plant and not obtained from a nutritious, natural plant grown on a farm or in the wild.

A recent study published in the *American Journal of Clinical Nutrition* showed that common doses of vitamin C—1,000 mg a day—can actually reduce oxygen uptake and significantly diminish endurance. Another recent study published in *Medicine & Science in Sports & Exercise* demonstrated that an antioxidant supplement, comprised of vitamins E and C, beta-carotene, zinc, and others in common use, did not prevent exercise-induced abnormalities, including inflammation, and may actually delay muscle recovery. But it's worth noting that the natural versions of these nutrients in a healthy diet will not cause these problems (and can significantly help runners). The fault is in the dietary supplement—and this includes the source (natural versus synthetic) and types of nutrients as well as the dosage. While the two studies cited here are contemporary ones, there are many others.

The most common nutrient that athletes are unable to obtain in a healthy diet is EPA from fish oil. The amount depends on the individual and his or her particular needs. Two to four capsules a day totaling about 1500 mg of EPA is an example of a typical dosage.

FOOD FREQUENCY

Once a runner decides to eat only healthy foods, there is another factor that is just as critical: frequency. Food intake is best spread out over the day.

The process of training and recovering often leaves runners ravenous and ready to chow down a big meal. This scenario has two drawbacks. First, getting this hungry during the day may mean the body is not burning sufficient fat for energy, lowering blood sugar and tapping into glycogen stores. Second, eating a large meal often results in less-than-adequate digestion and absorption of nutrients. Among the side-effects of poor digestion are bloating, excess gas, heartburn, nausea, diarrhea or constipation, and that feeling of fullness that can even linger into the next day's workout. But there is a way to have more consistent energy, feel better, and allow the body to get more nutrition out of each bite—eat smaller meals more frequently.

Without overeating, food frequency can help control insulin, burn more body fat, stabilize blood sugar and stress hormones, maintaining high energy, and reduce fat storage to the level of being lean.

This does not necessarily mean eating *more* food. Consider the runner who requires 3,000 calories a day. Instead of taking in these calories in say, three meals of a thousand calories each, consume six smaller meals of 500 calories. This might include breakfast, lunch and dinner with a mid-morning and mid-afternoon snack and a nutritious dessert in the evening. Basically, it means eating every two to four hours.

To get a runner ready for a 1:59 marathon, there is no single, recommended diet—except a healthy one devoid of all junk food. This includes the consumption of natural carbohydrates, proteins and fats at each meal. The total number of calories will naturally be determined by each runner's particular needs. As a general guideline, I would estimate that most marathoners require a diet that consists of about a third of each macronutrient (carbohydrate, protein and fat)—sufficient to obtain the necessary nutrients. This includes about ten servings of vegetables and fruits each day. Organic sources of fresh foods contain more nutrients, and without unhealthy chemicals.

NUTRITION

A healthy diet is absolutely essential for improving a runner's training and racing performance. The right foods help generate the following benefits: energy from stored body fat, highly efficient red muscle fibers, balanced blood sugar and hormones, high-quality red blood cells, and many other aspects of a healthy body and brain. Eating properly will enable a runner to stay injury-free, while training sufficiently in the overreaching state without breaking down or drifting into overtraining. Good nutrition improves running economy. It's a wonderful recipe for success.

CHAPTER 11

LIVE HIGH, TRAIN LOW

The beauty of Mammoth is the high-low.

—MEB KEFLEZIGHI, 2014 Boston Marathon
winner at age thirty-eight

Prior to the 1968 Summer Olympics in Mexico City, a number of athletes, coaches, and trainers expressed their concern about the effect of high altitude on competition. Mexico City sits at 7,350 feet, which is roughly more than one-and-one-third miles above sea level. Their worry focused on the perception that "the air is thinner" and would hamper performance.

"Thinner air" is a popular yet imprecise phrase, but what is really meant here is a decrease in barometric pressure as one gains altitude from sea level. While the amount of oxygen at Mexico City's elevation is the same as that found at sea level—all altitude levels contain 20.9 percent oxygen—the barometric pressure drops at higher elevation. It keeps decreasing the higher one goes. With less atmospheric pressure, oxygen uptake by the lungs is reduced, which means the body gets less of it.

But the International Olympic Committee thought otherwise, steadfastly claiming that competing at high altitude would have little, if any, effect on athletic performance. Instead, it recommended that athletes only had to spend a minimum of three or four days in Mexico City to adequately acclimate their bodies for the Games.

As it turned out, the IOC was proven quite wrong. Results from the Mexico Games were skewed in two opposite directions: much better and much worse. World records were broken in numerous track and field events. The most famous was Team USA's Bob Beamon's long jump of 29 feet, 2 ½ inches that was two feet longer than the previous world record. His teammate Lee Evans set the world record for 400 meters that lasted for almost twenty years. American sprinter Tommie Smith secured a world record in the 200 meters. Jim Hines, also of the US, became the first sprinter to break the 10-second barrier in the 100 meters (9.95 seconds).

If the Americans dominated the sprint events, the Kenyans took charge in the middle- and long-distance races, ushering in a new era of dominance that continues to this day. Kenyan runner Kipchoge Keino set a new Olympic record in the 1,500 meters (3:34.91), beating pre-race favorite Jim Ryun of the US by three seconds. Other than Keino, there were *no* world records established in races lasting longer than two-and-one-half minutes. Furthermore, many competitors from low-altitude regions raced far below expectations in distance events. Yet runners from high-altitude countries—Kenyans and Ethiopians—won at least one medal in all events 800 meters or longer.

The winning marathon time was a rather slow 2:20:26 by Ethiopian Mamo Wolde. (Earlier in the same Olympics, Wolde won silver in the 10,000, only .06 seconds behind Kenyan Temu Naftali.) Wolde's marathon time was more than three minutes ahead of the silver and bronze medalists (from low-altitude countries of Japan and New Zealand, respectively), and roughly eight minutes slower than Abebe Bikila's win at the 1964 Tokyo Games (held at sea level). Of the seventy-four starting marathoners at Mexico City, seventeen runners did not finish (including Bikila).

What accounted for this wide discrepancy in times at the Mexico Games? Why did sprinters benefit, becoming newly minted world-record holders? And why were the middle-distance and long-distance runners unable to establish world-record times? A simple explanation is that in the "thinner," less dense air, sprinting and jumping are easier due to lower air resistance, especially with less moisture. Hence, one can be more aerodynamic. But endurance running, which depends heavily on increased oxygen uptake, is instead restricted, raising heart rates and slowing the pace of runners.

Since the 1940s, anecdotal reports from athletes and coaches worldwide suggested that physiological benefits from altitude training could improve endurance for sea-level performance. When the Mexico City Games ended, altitude training became a much-studied discipline in scientific labs as exercise researchers, doctors, coaches, and athletes wanted to learn more about the subject. Yet it wasn't until 1985 that a key study on altitude training, "Living High—Training Low: Effect of Moderate-Altitude Acclimatization with Low-Altitude Training on Performance," was finally published in the *Journal of Applied Physiology*, by Dr. Benjamin Levine and Dr. James Stray-Gundersen, both from the Institute for Exercise and Environmental Medicine in Dallas, Texas. Their study revealed an optimal high-altitude approach to performance. They showed that over a four-week period, runners who lived at 8,200 feet but trained at a lower altitude (4,100 feet) improved their red blood cells, VO_2max and 5K race times compared to runners (the study's control group), who had trained at sea level. A third group, who trained *and* lived at the higher elevation, did *not* improve race times. Since then, hundreds of studies have been published in academic journals on altitude training, triggering a new trend in endurance sports: athletes need to get high!

Today, high-altitude living and training have become increasingly popular with professional runners, cyclists, and triathletes. But it must be emphasized that there are still many concerns and questions regarding the performance benefits, longevity of residency, and exact elevation. For example, if you are a top US distance runner, is it better to live in Boulder or Fort Collins, Colorado, each just over 5,000 feet, Flagstaff, Arizona, where one could run above 7,000 feet, or higher in Mammoth Lakes, California at 7,880 feet? And just how much time does one need to spend living at a higher elevation to begin noticing positive results? Finally, how does the body acclimate and what are these physiological changes?

Are endurance-athlete destinations in Colorado, Arizona, and California really necessary for those seeking faster race results? Yet there is no guarantee of improvement for all athletes who live at the higher elevation. In fact, there can be a decline in training and racing performance. Additionally, this decrease can happen with even the most highly trained athletes. There might be speed reductions of up to a minute-per-mile while going for an hour workout at the maximum aerobic heart rate. This is due to less oxygen taken out of the air and raising the heart rate significantly in order to get more blood to the muscles.

Clearly, *living* at higher altitudes can better prepare a runner to race faster at lower elevations, while competing at altitudes of about 2,000 feet can measurably impair oxygen consumption and reduce endurance race times. (Most of the popular big-city marathons are at sea level—and generally witness faster times by pro runners.) Since the atmosphere's *barometric pressure* is reduced, the body's ability to take oxygen out of the air is also reduced. The brain senses this change and makes an adaption through the production of more red blood cells by bone marrow, and even increasing lung size. These changes begin to take place immediately when arriving at higher altitudes.

The benefits of *living* at higher altitudes, typically between 4,000 and 8,000 feet, can result in a significant improvement of running economy, a reason it could speed up one's marathon times by up to four percent. But training at these levels will reduce one's pace and recovery times.

The ideal situation for endurance athletes, especially those seeking a 1:59 marathon, is as follows:

- Living at higher altitude, 7,000–8,000 feet
- Training at lower elevations, 4,000 feet or lower
- Racing at the lowest altitude (sea level or below) produces faster times.

East Africans who reside at higher altitudes have been dominating endurance sports since the late 1960s. Coming down to lower elevations to race provides an obvious advantage of more red blood cells to bring additional oxygen to muscles. But this effect is not because they train at high elevation, which may actually take away from their great racing abilities. The larger question is: how much faster could they run if their training took place at lower altitudes, where daily recovery is also better, while living at higher elevations? It is certainly possible that we would have seen a 1:59 marathon by now if many of the top Kenyan runners lived high, trained low.

The physiological mechanisms behind the benefits of altitude living begin with the body's production of EPO (erythropoietin). This hormone stimulates the making of more red blood cells, which can then carry additional oxygen to muscles. EPO is produced by the kidneys, and can also improve brain function, and increase iron absorption from the intestines, which is necessary to make new, higher quality red blood cells.

External sources of EPO are used in medicine for patients with kidney and intestinal diseases, and certain cancers. In the 1990s, blood doping with synthetic EPO in endurance sports such as professional cycling began, but its detection in athletes was not possible until 2000. Today, EPO can be detected in both blood and urine, and is a regular part of drug testing.

In addition to positive changes in the quality and quantity of red blood cells, other important benefits can occur with high-altitude living. Improvements in the aerobic system can be significant. These include better circulation in aerobic muscles, enabling better blood flow, increases in myoglobin (the red pigment in aerobic muscle fibers that can improve their function), and more aerobic enzymes to boost fat burning.

However, regardless of whether the elevation is 5,000 or 8,000 feet, or somewhere in between, a runner must train by sub-maximum heart rate and not by pace, otherwise the risk of overtraining increases. Slower training paces will exist until acclimatization occurs, which could take up to two weeks for athletes not used to higher attitudes. But even at elevations above 4,000 feet, slower maximum aerobic paces compared to sea level will prevail.

Another important factor regarding living at altitude, even when training at lower elevations, is timing the descent to where the race is held. Traveling to sea level two weeks before race day may be the ideal situation. This immediately results in an improvement in oxygen uptake, and with higher amounts of red blood cells, better performance can follow.

Not all research has found that athletes who live at altitude are able to increase their red-blood cell counts and improve performance. This could be due to nutritional and genetic factors.

While science has yet to identify any specific genes in East African distance runners that give them a directly, measurable advantage, one possible explanation for their consistent performances could be from living and training at altitude. High-altitude locations in Kenya's Rift Valley and elsewhere, including Ethiopia, is where many of these superior distance runners call home or spend much of the year. Populations evolved in these environments for several million years—sufficient time for nature to make genetic changes. But having lean legs, including thin ankles and calves, are not enough to ensure optimal running economy. The body must still be properly nurtured with the right nutrients. Diet might help explain the disparity between those runners who benefit from altitude and those who experience a decrease in performance.

Many East African champions came from a life at high elevations, but only a relatively small number of people from these regions have become great runners. In fact, it's mostly concentrated among the Nandi-speaking tribes of Kenya's Rift Valley, or Kalenjin people, who number less than five million. The vast majority of Kenyan running stars, men as well as women, are Kalenjin.

Another possible reason that explains why a Kenyan or Ethiopian marathon running champion hasn't yet gone 1:59 might be traced to nutritional imbalances, which is quite common in developing countries. One important example of this dietary imbalance is iron status. The ability to make more quality red-blood cells, even with EPO production, can be reduced when iron levels are too low. Despite the body's adaptation to living at altitude, which can result in improved intestinal absorption of iron by three to four times, many athletes are still too low in iron. This is usually due to diet inadequacy rather

185

than a regular need for an iron supplement. Consuming a healthy diet, especially foods high in useable iron such as red meat, will provide the body with sufficient amounts of this mineral to make appropriate levels of quality red cells in response to altitude living. (Vegetable sources of iron are poorly absorbed.)

One warning for all runners if an iron supplement is necessary: care must be taken when considering taking one. This is especially true in doses above 10 mg, since iron supplements can cause significant free-radical stress, and even physical damage to the intestines.

Folic acid status could also have a significant effect on the production of both EPO and red blood cells. This nutrient is often low in runners due to an insufficient daily consumption of vegetables such as spinach, beets, Brussels sprouts and broccoli; there are even higher levels of folic acid found in lentils, beef, and turkey. Runners who rely on a dietary supplement for their folic acid needs may be surprised to know that this vitamin form is usually synthetic, and for many people the body is often unable to utilize it.

Other nutritional factors can significantly influence the effectiveness of living high. EPO production requires adequate protein intake, and can be impaired by chronic inflammation. To properly regulate inflammation requires balancing dietary fats, and obtaining sufficient omega-3 fats from fish oil, which also impact the quality of red blood cells produced at altitude.

To ensure the maximum benefits of "live high, train low," a runner should have his blood tested before going to altitude, or while he or she is living there. Here's is a short list of what should be measured:

- A complete blood count (CBC) to monitor red-cell count, hemoglobin, and hematocrit gives a more complete picture of physiological benefits.

- Testing levels of iron, ferritin, folic acid, vitamin B12, and other nutrients as necessary provides information to ensure a runner has the raw materials to obtain optimal benefits of being at altitude.
- The C-reactive protein (CRP) test can help rule out chronic inflammation.
- Although usually unnecessary except in difficult cases (such as those who don't respond to high altitude living), EPO can also be assessed through a blood test.

In addition, there is an increased risk of dehydration at higher elevations because of lower humidity and increased loss of water from the body. Consuming small amounts of water throughout the day can help maintain proper hydration.

Living at altitude can suppress one's appetite, often leading to lower nutrient intake. This can result in a reduction of body weight, some of which is water, but most of the weight may be muscle loss, and in some cases reduced muscle function. This makes meal planning even more essential when living at altitude.

HIGH-ALTITUDE CHAMBERS

Runners can temporarily experience living at low and high altitudes, respectively, with the use of mild hyperbaric and hypobaric chambers. They can also be used at any elevation. These can potentially provide the same benefits as living high. (Hyperbaric refers to higher barometric pressure, while hypobaric is lower pressure.)

Mild hyperbaric chambers can simulate low altitude because their high barometric pressure raises oxygen uptake, even without the addition of extra oxygen. A runner can use the chamber for about forty-five minutes each day following a training session to help speed recovery. The oxygen uptake's elevating effects occur immediately.

Hypobaric chambers simulate higher altitude, sometimes up to 18,000 feet, because they create low pressure, stimulating the production of EPO. This exposes a runner to a high-altitude environment while at rest—napping, reading, and relaxing, or sleeping through the night. It provides the convenience of living high while at lower altitudes (even sea level).

Hypobaric chambers are large and heavy, and not as portable as the small, inflatable, mild hyperbaric chambers. The expense of these devices has limited their widespread use, with costs in the thousands of dollars for newer units.

Just like living at high altitude, the use of these chambers is basically a "natural" form of blood doping. The World Anti-Doping Agency even considered placing "artificially-induced hypoxic conditions" on the 2007 Prohibited List of Substances/Methods to avoid competitive advantages acquired by athletes who used them, but in the end did not. They are still legal to use.

SUNSHINE: HELP FROM ABOVE

Another environmental benefit of living high is that the body can be exposed to more sunlight. Low moisture and cleaner air, typical of high elevations, allow much more sun to reach the body. This can provide optimal levels of one of the body's most important nutrients: vitamin D.

For millions of years, the human body's relationship with the sun was critically important for two primary reasons. One is that it increased our production of a *prohormone* referred to as vitamin D, which helps muscles and other bodily systems work better. It is through these and other actions that vitamin D can affect running economy.

Vitamin D helps control inflammation and immunity, improves brain and hormone function, regulates calcium absorption and utilization, and promotes the work of thousands of genes. It can improve muscle function and avoid unwanted loss of muscle, prevent stress fractures, help with training and racing recovery, and prevent more serious health problems including many forms of cancer. Normal vitamin D levels may also prevent sunburn during long training runs and races.

But inadequate vitamin D is common among athletes, especially runners who might only train early in the morning or in the late afternoon or evening hours. They then spend the rest of the daylight hours indoors.

For runners who don't live full time in sunny environments, it's critical to obtain adequate vitamin D from sun exposure during the warmer summer months to build stores of vitamin D for winter use.

How much sun and for how long depends on each runner's individual needs, with skin color, geographic location and season being key factors. Even fair-skinned athletes are at risk of low vitamin D, even though most can easily obtain it with short amounts of sunshine. The daily exposure of the arms and legs to sunlight for twenty to thirty minutes may be sufficient—more in northern climates and less when closer to the equator. The best times of the day to obtain vitamin D are between the hours of 10 a.m. and 3 p.m. In a healthy runner, this amount of sun can produce 5,000 to 10,000 units of vitamin D, which is not excessive. Interestingly, you can't overdose on vitamin D from the sun like you can from dietary supplements.

As sunlight tans the skin, longer periods of sun exposure will be needed to obtain vitamin D. That's because those with darker skin, which blocks sunlight, require even more sun exposure to obtain the same amount of vitamin D. This is especially important for those in more northern and extreme southern climates. Those with the darkest skin require the most sun exposure to maintain adequate levels of vitamin D. This is most easily accomplished at higher altitudes in warmer climates, but more difficult elsewhere.

As the levels of vitamin D rise and normalize, the risk of sunburn diminishes, even in those with well-tanned white skin. It's important to balance minimizing overexposure with obtaining enough sun to allow for sufficient vitamin D production.

While research indicates that blood levels of vitamin D around 50 ng/ml are associated with peak athletic performance, a surprising number of runners have much lower levels. The reasons for this deficiency include the following:

1. Using sunscreen that blocks the vitamin D–producing ultraviolet B (UVB) waves of the sun.
2. Wearing protective clothing, especially materials that block UVB waves.
3. Training early and later in the day, when vitamin D–producing sun exposure is significantly reduced.
4. Darker skin. Even many light-skinned athletes have accumulated enough sun to darken their skin to the point that it reduces their ability to obtain vitamin D from sun exposure. As a result, they need to be in the sun longer to obtain the same amount of D.
5. Those with too high or too low body fat may be unable to release and utilize stored vitamin D.

6. Athletes living at more extreme latitudes, such as northern Europe and Canada, and southern Australia and South America, have significantly less sun exposure throughout the year.

Without sufficient sun exposure throughout the year to maintain adequate vitamin D levels, supplementation may be necessary.

VITAMIN D SUPPLEMENTS

The best dietary supplement for vitamin D is cod liver oil because it contains the most efficient form called D3, or cholecalciferol. The vitamin D2 form (ergocalciferol) is obtained from plants but less effective, and a common source in most other dietary supplements. D2 is also used in fortified packaged foods (most of which is junk food), and almost always contains very small amounts.

Some athletes have dangerously low blood levels of vitamin D, and even modest amounts of supplementation may not correct it. In these cases, a healthcare practitioner may prescribe high doses to correct this problem (such as 50,000 IU a day or more for the first week)—amounts that must be carefully monitored with blood tests to avoid toxicity while ensuring vitamin D levels return to normal. (Indications of toxicity may include fatigue, constipation, forgetfulness, nausea, and vomiting.)

Sunshine and the Brain

Sunlight also helps the brain. The eyes are part of the brain, and seeing natural sunlight can help us think and feel better. No, not staring into the sun, but allowing the eyes to be exposed to natural outdoor light—without contact lenses, eyeglasses, sunglasses and windows, all of which block the beneficial rays.

The human eye contains photosensitive cells in its retina. Stimulation of these cells, from the blue unseen spectrum of sunlight can help runners in at least two ways:

- Stimulation of the brain's hypothalamus region and pituitary gland, which is important for sleeping and recovery, hormone regulation, and when adjusting to jet lag.
- The brain's pineal gland benefits directly from sun stimulation by producing melatonin. This important hormone, actually made during dark hours, protects the skin. In addition, melatonin is a powerful antioxidant, critical for proper sleep and intestinal function, and can help prevent depression. (Taking aspirin can reduce melatonin production.)

All these effects on the eyes can influence how you feel the next morning, helping you get out of bed for your early run. The transition from sleep to waking up requires the effects of the body's adrenal glands, influenced by the brain's hypothalamus and pituitary. (Many don't experience these benefits until their morning coffee kicks in.) Once up, exposure to morning sunlight helps raise body temperature to normal (after a slight reduction during sleep), and then warms up the body. In addition, numerous brain activities including increased alertness and better cognition can help mood and vitality. In short, if you want to get a bit more benefit from your workout, let the sun shine.

Just as you should avoid excess sun exposure, you should obviously keep away from the uncomfortable glare from the sun, which might indicate *too much* light is entering the eye. Normal exposure to daily light, however, should not cause damage because the body is protected by antioxidants and other nutrients that are part of a healthy diet.

Inside lighting may provide some eye stimulation if the light bulbs are the full-spectrum type. But it won't take the place of a regular habit of getting the morning sun into unshielded eyes for only a few seconds.

THE NEED TO SWEAT IT

The human body is built to run dry—our physiology is naturally equipped to handle that environment. For several million years, northeast Africa is where humans ran to survive, hunting much larger animals by outrunning them over long distances. One factor allowing us to function so well in dry weather, especially on race day, is our sweat mechanism.

Sweating is important for cooling the body. It prevents too much of an elevation in temperature that can slow one's pace. But sweat must quickly evaporate to be most efficient at this task. A non-dry race location, where more humid air reduces sweat evaporation, would not be ideal for heat regulation, and therefore not the best environment for a 1:59 marathon. (Heat loss also occurs by convection—the movement of air across the skin.)

Humans evolved with much less body hair than most other mammals. This helped us naturally regulate body temperature. So covering the body with clothing, even a racing singlet, during the marathon, could become an issue. The racers vying for 1:59 may best forego their sponsors' logos and run without singlets to avoid trapping heat. Clothing can interfere with heat regulation like a coat of fur, although certainly not as much. But every second counts when the goal is 1:59. The hair on one's head should also be kept very short for the same reason.

Instead of living *and* training high, as many elite East African runners already do, there should be more of an effort to recalibrate this way of thinking. But it's hard to argue with success, that is, until something new beckons. Imagine brand-new running camps for elite runners springing up in high-altitude areas that also allow quick and easy access to training at lower altitudes. So when race day does arrive, and it happens to be a non-humid one, and the venue is at sea level, the 1:59 marathon may be just a step away for the well-prepared runner who lived high and trained low.

Chapter 12

Women

I'll never do that again!

> —Grete Waitz, after winning the first of nine
> consecutive New York City Marathons

I have waited until now to discuss women marathoners. Are they also capable of going 1:59 like their male counterparts? The short answer is probably not yet, at least in the near future. Conceivably, women have the necessary endurance and speed. They are indeed physiologically capable of going sub-two hours. But before that ever happens, quite a lot has to change regarding how women pro runners approach their training and racing. It might be best for most women to train in a way that optimally matches their biological strengths, rather than follow the training practices of top male marathoners.

Let's start with Paula Radcliffe, an amazingly talented runner from England, who is the current world-record holder in the marathon. In 2003, she blazed to 2:15:25 in the London Marathon. Radcliffe's time would have been a world-best for men right up until the year 1958. In the same London race, the men's winner, an Ethiopian by the name of Gezahegne Abera went 2:07:56. Radcliffe's impressive showing placed her sixteenth overall. But nearly seven-and-one-half minutes can seem like an eternity in the marathon.

One study compared the times of the top five women and men finishers in seven of the world's largest marathons over a 12-year period (1997 to 2009). Dr. Sandra Hunter, of Marquette University in Milwaukee, Wisconsin, found times for these women finishers to be 10 to 12 percent behind the top men. This percentage gap would seem to suggest that a woman marathoner might not run 1:59 until men are battling it out in the 1:50 zone. For many, this scenario might seem iffy, more like the stuff of science fiction. Yet it is not implausible to consider these sub-two hour times, for men and women, respectively, as potentially happening one day in the future. Women marathoners will—and should—get faster.

For example, in 2014, Rita Jeptoo of Kenya became a three-time winner at the Boston Marathon by going 2:18:57, which beat the course record by almost two full minutes. Finishing twenty-first overall, she ran the twenty-fourth mile in 4:49. She beat her last year's winning time by almost eight minutes. Yet despite Jeptoo's stellar performance in Boston as the eighth fastest women's time ever recorded on any marathon course, no woman runner has been able to lower Radcliffe's eleven-year-old world record. Since 2003, however, the men's world record has been broken four times.

The marathon is a men's race, created by men long ago in honor of a fallen hero from antiquity. Ever since the first modern Olympics when the marathon became the gold standard for distance running, men have had a long time to figure out how best to train for the race based on their masculine strengths, which include muscle power and testosterone.

MARATHON WOMEN

Women's participation in running events, from 5Ks to marathons (and now ultras), did not begin to show an increase in numbers until the 1970s. Today, in the US, approximately 40 percent of all marathon finishers are women. In half-marathons, which is the fastest growing sector of racing, 60 percent of all finishers are women.

But the road to running hasn't been easy for women. Nor did it occur overnight. For some historical perspective, let's look at the recent past. Several weeks before the start of the 1996 Atlanta Olympic Games, an essay appeared in the Sunday Magazine of the *New York Times* whose headline read "How the Women Won." The piece opened with these two provocative paragraphs:

When the modern Olympics began in Athens in 1896, one dismissive tradition carried over from the ancient games. All 245 athletes from 14 nations who competed in Athens were men. Women were expected to lend their applause, not their athletic skills. Olympic historians now believe that two women ran the marathon course near or during the Games. If so, the organizers were unimpressed. Distance running by women was thought to be un-ladylike, a violation of natural law. The common wisdom held that a woman was not physiologically capable of running mile after mile; that she wouldn't be able to bear children; that her uterus would fall out; that she might grow a mustache; that she was a man, or wanted to be one.

When six women collapsed after the 800-meter race at the 1928 Amsterdam Olympics, an alarmist account in the New York Times *said that, "even this distance makes too great a call on feminine strength." The* London Daily Mail *carried admonitions from doctors that women who participated in such "feats of endurance" would "become old too soon." The 800-meter race was discontinued. For 32 years, until the 1960 Rome Olympics, women would run no race longer than 200 meters.*

That gender restriction eventually changed, but it wasn't a simple thing to shake off tradition's chastity belt. A small group of old men ran the Olympics. They had even older-fashioned views about women and sports unless it involved "ladylike" activities such as swimming, diving, ice-skating, and gymnastics.

Then along came late-Sixties' pioneers such as Kathrine Switzer who ran the Boston Marathon in 1967 when women were officially prohibited. Switzer's trailblazing performance that year made news headlines around the world after a photo captured race director Jock Semple storming onto the course as he tried to grab hold of her, yelling, "Get the hell out of my race and give me those numbers!" But Switzer's boyfriend, a burly hammer thrower, who was running by her side, shoved Semple off to the side. Afterwards, the American Athletic Union barred women from all competition with male runners. Women were not allowed to enter the Boston marathon officially until five years later. Yet the tide had changed. And women started showing up at races across the country.

Eventually, Switzer, who won the 1974 New York City Marathon, competed at Boston six times, finishing second in 1975 with a PR of 2:51. She also helped launched the Avon International Running Circuit of women's-only races in twenty-seven countries.

Women's running greatly benefited from the passage of Title IX in 1972 as part of the Education Act—the amendment outlawed gender-based discrimination at colleges that received US federal funds. The new law triggered an explosion of college athletic scholarships for young women, which, in turn encouraged more girls to play sports in high school. One was Joan Benoit Samuelson, of Maine, who took the gold in the first Olympic marathon for women held at the Los Angeles Games in 1984 (her time was 2:24). She ran track in high school. She even won the 1975 state championship in the mile—but it was also the longest distance that a high school girl was then allowed to run in a track meet.

Today, it is not uncommon for elite women runners to keep pace with men.

In races longer than the marathon, women have outperformed men in winning overall. Ultra-marathoner Ann Trason has won several 150-mile events outright. In 2002, Pam Reed was the first woman to become the overall winner of the Badwater Ultramarathon in Death Valley, a remarkable feat of endurance that she repeated in 2003.

In most areas of the world, such as in East Africa, the cultural or gender gap between men and women is much wider than found in the West. Yet like the male East Africans, women runners from this region have shown dominance in almost all the large-city marathons with hefty cash purses. Since 2009, a Kenyan or Ethiopian has won the women's division in the last four New York City Marathons (the race was cancelled in 2012 due to Hurricane Sandy.) At the Boston Marathon, a Kenyan or Ethiopian woman has won sixteen of the past eighteen races. (Russian women won the two other times.) And in the Olympics, Kenyan or Ethiopian women have won six of the 24 medals in the marathon since 1984 (compared to nine for the men during the same period).

Like they do when the topic is the dominance of East African male runners, many in the media view professional Kenyan and Ethiopian women runners in a similar fashion. Articles are filled with talk about genetics, skinny legs, and so on. There is no denying that Kenyan and Ethiopian women work physically hard and had very active childhoods. If they are some of the best endurance runners in the world right now, it's due to many of the same reasons that help explain the East African men's success. Their living and training environment develops their bodies better than most of their competition in the West. This includes growing up barefoot, with its many developmental benefits. Living at high elevations helps too, with more red blood cells and better circulation.

There are also social and economic factors. A successful career in running, with prize money and sponsorships, offers talented women athletes an escape from a poor rural life; and in turn, it's how they can help their families and communities. Running is imprinted in their lives from an early age. Many run several miles to school every day, and then back home. Cross-country race are popular among young girls who typically run barefoot.

CLOSING THE GENDER GAP

It wasn't all that long ago, when sports doctors, coaches, and trainers attempted to narrow the gender performance gap between men and women through artificial means. Sports officials in East Germany and the former Soviet Union condoned the use of testosterone therapy for their women athletes. Yes, they got stronger, more muscular, and set new world records, but they also began to look and sound like men. Those days are thankfully past.

Instead, there are natural ways for women to close the performance gap with men. Most importantly, their progress would be enhanced if they focused on training as women, and not as men. Viewed solely from a biological standpoint, there are noticeable differences between male and female runners. Whereas elite male runners might have VO_2max values upward of around 85, top women runners average about 10 percent less. This is due to lower hemoglobin concentrations, and as a result, less oxygen gets to the muscles.

Men also have higher levels of testosterone, which is a primary reason that they have more muscle mass and greater strength.

For the same body size, women have smaller lungs, and narrower airways. But women can adapt better, compensating well for what appears to be these apparent disadvantages. For example, studies show that their diaphragm muscle, which pulls air in and out of the lungs, is more resistant to fatigue compared to men. With smaller lungs and narrower airways, the respiratory muscles in women have evolved over time to better withstand fatigue, which is very important for training and racing.

Studies have also shown that a female athlete's muscular system has greater endurance capacity than men's. Despite women having less muscle mass, this endurance advantage seems to offset their reduced strength relative to men. Women may experience less physical fatigue in their bodies than men. The reasons for this benefit may be better blood flow in women, and improved muscle metabolism regarding the use of body fat for energy.

Another example is found when measuring the quadricep muscles. There is an overall greater relative activation of these muscles during fatigue in women compared to men. Researchers are not quite sure why this is the case, but less "fatigueability" is obviously beneficial in training as it can result in faster recovery. And it can help racing.

While men naturally make more testosterone, women have more estrogen. This female hormone helps the brain resist fatigue, along with other benefits. Additionally, estrogen protects muscles from exercise-induced damage, which may be one of the reasons women burn more fat than men. Muscles that fatigue less function better for longer periods, and recover more quickly from training and racing. But the estrogen factor in female runners is nearly lost if overtraining occurs.

A higher level of fat burning in women can help better develop their aerobic base, countering the reduced VO_2max and testosterone. Finally, by burning more body fat during an endurance competition like the marathon, women's supply of liver and muscle glycogen can outlast that of men.

Other factors regarding women distance runners are as follows:

- The reduced hemoglobin in women can be offset with high-altitude living while training at lower elevations.
- Women have shorter Achilles tendons than men, which can be advantageous in generating more impact energy from the foot and leg's elastic recoil mechanism.
- Due to their smaller size, women should tolerate hot and humid racing conditions better than men, making them less susceptible to overheating.

In the book, *The Natural Superiority of Women,* author and anthropologist Ashley Montague discusses the scientific evidence supporting the long-time claim that women are biologically superior to men, in most of the ways other than physical strength. In addition to quicker recovery from workouts, this also means improved immune systems for better health. On average, women live several years more than men. Women also appear to have a greater knack when it comes time to coordinate the different areas of the brain necessary during a race—something that could mean increased running economy.

By leveraging these physiological attributes, the top women runners can go a lot faster. This will narrow the gender gap. In his classic book, *The Lore of Running,* Dr. Tim Noakes writes, "Armed with these advantages, women are in a position to do endurance feats previously considered by men to be impossible." We won't see a woman running 1:59 before a man does. But they won't be that far behind, either.

TRAINING LIKE WOMEN CHAMPIONS

As I have often personally witnessed throughout my coaching career, one of the main obstacles that women encounter is their desire to work out like the men—high mileage weeks, hard training sessions, and adapting the male-centric jock philosophy of "no pain no gain." One clearly obvious problem with this unhealthy approach to training, which relies more on muscle strength, is that overtrained women are in greater potential of becoming injured. Overtraining diminishes women's advantages, and the resulting reductions in estrogen are usually significant. This can trigger bone and muscle impairments, and wide array of hormone and neurological imbalances that are all part of the overtraining syndrome.

Women have lower maximum heart rates compared to men, as one recent study showed. But the 180 Formula still works great for them since it is not based on resting or maximum heart rates, but rather one's level of fitness and health.

So if a woman can theoretically run a 1:59 marathon, when will it happen? No one can know or predict with any certainty. But don't assume the current 10 to 12 percent lag time with male marathoners will continue indefinitely. Instead, expect women's world-record times in the coming years to start decreasing at a faster rate than men's.

When a male runner finally goes 1:59, will this have a spillover effect on women's performance and times? One of the things that we learned from Roger Bannister's 3:59 mile is that women don't sit idly by and watch from the sidelines. Only twenty-three days after Bannister broke the men's four-minute barrier, Diane Leather, also of England, broke the women's five-minute mile time in 4:59.

Finally, the men's mile record is currently 3:43.13, set in 1999 by Hicham el Guerrouj of Morocco. The women's mile record is 4:12.56, established by Svetlana Masterkova of Russia in 1996. While the women's world-record mile mark fell by an overall greater amount since 1954 (47 seconds vs. 16 seconds), the current performance gap between top male and female milers is still within the 10 to 12 percent gender range of elite runners. With improved training, it's entirely possible that a woman miler will someday go 3:59. Perhaps it might happen right around the time that a woman marathoner goes 1:59. Both women runners might even appear on the same cover of *Time* magazine's "Person of the Year" issue.

Chapter 13

Brain

The idea that the harder you work, the better you're going to be is just garbage. The greatest improvement is made by the man or woman who works most intelligently.

—Bill Bowerman, co-founder of Nike and
legendary track coach

What is the brain's role in running a marathon? As the elite runner relentlessly pushes his body toward the precipice of complete exhaustion, what are the conscious (and unconscious) thought processes inside his head? Heroically warding off fatigue, can he maintain the fast pace and blot out the pain? Do emotions intrude, and if so, how do they change over the course of running 26.2 miles? To answers these questions, let's begin by taking a brief fictional detour.

What is it like to run a 1:59 marathon from the subjective perspective of the athlete's brain? Our journey begins at the race start where our runner is lined up with two dozen pro distance-running specialists. Each has previously run the marathon under 2:05 or faster in the past year.

Race day is finally here. The start is just several minutes away. Though it feels like it will be eons. Time is distorted. It's as if everything is slowing down. Or rather not happening, until the gun goes off. Then I know everything will become a rapid blur of motion.

My brain and body know the race plan well. They are a team. Rather, "we" are a team. Both coach and athlete. Each doing its important share. We have rehearsed this routine for thousands of hours in training—how to run at a 4:35-per-mile pace for twenty-six miles—but without actually going the entire distance. The longest training run was two-and-a-half hours, but at a slightly slower pace. I only hope today's final miles won't be too painful, and that my body has enough energy for a final kick.

I will be racing against the clock and my body's pain threshold. It's up to the brain to manage both race pace and pain. This well-protected small organ might only weigh three pounds, but it contains 30 billion neurons. The brain is an energy hog, taking 20 percent of the oxygen that I inhale and the same percentage of blood that my heart pumps.

But my heart now seems to be beating faster than my regular resting rate of 35 beats per minute. I need to take a few deep breaths to slow it down.

I imagine the other runners to my immediate left and right are experiencing the same pre-race anxiety. No one is talking or looking at one another. Several appear to be lightly moving back and forth on the balls of their feet. Others remain stationary. I have an image of my own feet being stuck in cement. Not a good sign. Need to think of something else. But what?

There's a dreamlike quality to my thoughts. Despite the body's high sympathetic state of readiness, my brain seems caught inside an alpha-state of consciousness. It's like a runner's trance, a heightened awareness. But the runner's trance is not the same as a runner's high. That will come later, much later . . . once the race is over.

Mentally drifting along this altered state, the image of my feet encased in cement disappears. I now feel as if I'm floating several feet above the starting line. The din of the crowd of spectators reminds me of the sound of ocean waves crashing onto the beach. I think back to all those barefoot runs on the sandy dunes in one instantaneous, indistinct blur.

Wait . . . reality check. The present. My body feels tingly, on high alert. It's fight or flight. I look down at my palms. They are sweaty and feel hot, despite the early morning's cool temperature. Having received a message from my brain's auditory centers, the motor cortex is prepping the right index finger, which is gently resting on the little button of the Garmin watch. I lean forward. I'm poised. I'm ready.

The gun sounds. It seems louder than normal because of the charged state my body is in. Even the bones in my legs feel the crack of the gun going off. I press the watch's start button, but my feet seem not to move. Then, in another instant, my brain takes over, commanding my right leg to move across the starting line. The left leg obediently follows without deliberate prompting. My body feels like a rocket ship leaving the launch pad.

I am off. My legs power forward with smooth intensity.I can thank the brain for making these first few hundred yards go without much difficulty or muscle stiffness. Chemical signals are being passed from the brain to my legs at seemingly supersonic speeds.

The first-mile marker arrives. I shoot a glance down at my watch: 4:32. Okay, three seconds too fast, and probably due to the sympathetic drive—the nervous system's chemical surge from the hypothalamus, located deep in the middle of the brain. Two runners have pulled ahead and are now a dozen or so yards ahead of me. They are using too much glycogen for such an early surge.

Now that my body has had its first-mile fling, it's critical to settle into a groove of maximum running economy. There's a small clump of runners on both sides. Our footsteps appear to be striking the ground at the same time.

Mile two comes, and I have "slowed" to 4:37. My race pace has been naturally restored. This has occurred because the brain's cortex has gathered information from the body, and with this data, it has been busy calculating with the power of a roomful of supercomputers, all the nearly infinite variables involving the different contractions and relaxations of each of the millions of muscle fibers in my body. It combines this data with ongoing information from tendons and joints about the quality of the gait, and how much fuel from body fat and sugar is being used.

The two lead runners have widened their lead to nearly fifty yards. Am I running too slowly? The rational part of the brain does not allow this worry to take charge; instead, it determines that my pace is just fine.

Each foot strike is minutely processed and analyzed by the brain, making sure there's no wasted energy on ground impact and the elastic-recoil effect is efficient. Meanwhile, the cerebellum coordinates with both the motor centers high up in the brain, and the brainstem at the bottom, to synchronize my breathing, heart rate, and stride. The result is three steps for each inhalation, then four more while exhaling.

There is no room for my limbic system's emotions to interfere or cloud the present. I have laser focus, though I seem to be running on autopilot as I continue to cover ground. My body is leaning slightly forward, head completely upright, eyes straight ahead, with arms swinging to help the torso rotate just right.

The five-mile mark appears right on schedule at 22:53. Yes! I sneak a glance of a volunteer's face while passing the water station. She looked surprised that I didn't grab the cup she was holding. No need for additional hydration in a race of this short duration. It would only slow me down. Each and every second matters and must be accounted for.

The next five miles have a hypnotic-like regularity, as if my body is along for the ride. But that's not true either. It's only my brain doing its job.

Ten miles and everything has so far gone according to our pre-race strategy. Elapsed time: 45:47. Even in the cool morning, my body temperature has been rising and I'm covered in a light sheen of sweat. At the 11-mile mark, I impulsively reach for a cup of water from a volunteer at the aid station, and dump it on my head. The sensation of cool water on my hot bare scalp feels soothing.

At the halfway point, I peek down at the Garmin. It flashes 59:59. This makes me want to smile, but not enough for the skin around my mouth to move, so it does not show. I continue to stare straight ahead, not seeing any of the crowd or hearing its loud roar. Only two runners are now near me, one to the immediate left and another slightly behind. We are gradually reeling in the two lead runners whose gap has dwindled to five yards.

The brain knows just how much more running—and at what pace— is required for the second half of the race. It is still making the rapid-fire computations on how much fuel, water, and electrolytes are needed, as well as the level of muscle, tendon, ligament, bone and joint stress that can be tolerated without significant damage to the body.

Then, seemingly out of nowhere, the brain's conscious cortex sends out a distress signal, readying the body for another change in response to the onset of accumulated fatigue in the muscles. This change results in a slight shortening of the stride. The cadence increases proportionately. As both changes are implemented, I try to stay relaxed. Or as relaxed as one's body can be considering that the pace is one of the fastest ever run for this distance. My brain offers assistance by presenting a mental picture—a snapshot—of my body crossing the finish line.

I have now caught up to the two lead runners as they have both slowed. One falls back and out of sight, the other stays with me. But he appears to be struggling, his gait looking almost ragged. And he's breathing hard.

Mile 15 passes in 1:08:41. Fatigue has spread across my entire body, and it's especially felt in my legs. The fatigue manifests itself in a dull, generalized pain. Now the war of attrition is on. The enemy forces are exhaustion and suffering.

Mile 19 must have passed. Concentrating on maintaining a smooth, natural gait is getting much more difficult. It's up to the brain not to shirk from its duty of keeping my speed fast and fluid.

Mile 20 is here . . . 1:31:35. Excellent. Still on target. Can't falter now.

The urge to wet my head again with water is strong, so I grab a cup. But I quickly realize it's not in my hand, I missed it. Okay, just wait for the next station.

Just before mile 22, the general pain worsens. My entire body is hurting. It's on fire. Then all of a sudden, a different kind of pain appears. There's a sharp, stinging sensation in my right hip. It's as if an ice pick is being jabbed into the joint. Many areas of the brain had been monitoring this region and now must act without delay. The cause was a minor imbalance between certain weakening psoas muscle fibers and a tightening of others in the hamstring. The gait was affected and the hip joint's movement became imprecise.

The brain tries to correct the problem. The motor center on the left side of the cortex, which controls the right side of my body, sends messages to nearby muscle fibers in the psoas to help out. The quadriceps compensates too, by contracting slightly more with each flexion of the hip. Fortunately, within a quarter mile, adequate muscle balance is restored. The hip pain diminishes sufficiently, although it still lingers. The gait is only mildly impaired.

At mile 24, another quick cup of water sloshed on my head. It will be my last. I am now running alone. Two cops on large motorcycles are just in front. I hear but don't see the thumping helicopter overhead.

Mile 25. Time is 1:54:31. I do my best to ignore the discomfort in the right hip and the cumulative effect of body-wide fatigue. My brain is sacrificing a lot—blood sugar is diminished, and glycogen stores are rapidly dwindling. Basically, my gas tank is practically empty. But I nonetheless feel that I still have enough energy left for a strong finishing kick.

Mile 26. I can't spare any excess energy to even check the time on the watch. I am running on pure animal instinct, and buoyed by the thunderous roar and cheering of spectators.

The moment of truth has arrived for a final kick. The brain makes one more maximum effort to go faster. What's left of my sympathetic drive produces a tsunami of stress hormones. I have never felt this much hurt in all the years of running.

The finish line tape draws closer. Two hundred yards, then one hundred, then 50, 25, 10. Then it happens. I reach the tape. As my chest pushes through the ripped, fluttering paper band covered by the race sponsor's logo, my legs give out and I fall to the ground. Breathing rapidly and barely able to move, I roll over onto my non-aching left side and look at the large timing display stationed next to the finish line. I only can see the first three digits of the two-foot high clock. "1:59" . . . That's all my brain needs to process for the moment. Medical personnel crowd around me, I am unable to feel much excitement, just a sense of disbelief and awe. Then, a flurry of new sensations suddenly appears to rise up from the base of my spine, and travels further north into my head. Finally freed from its 119-minute captivity, the brain's hitherto tightly constrained limbic system releases a surge of emotions. Tears begin to roll down my cheeks, mixing with sweat. I made marathon history. Wait, allow me to correct myself. We made marathon history. Brain and body. Together as a winning team.

Nature has provided us with a magnificent gift: the human brain. As our intelligence developed over several million years, the human species went from being primitive hunters and gatherers relying on simple stone tools for survival to populations built around highly complex societies living in cities. During the past century, science and technology have accelerated to the point where it's nearly impossible to comprehend just how far we have progressed from our Paleolithic past that ended roughly 10,000 years ago. Yet much of our genetic past still remains within us, intact and undisturbed, and ready to be called into action. I am referring to our natural ability to run long distances. Other species don't have this quality in warm or moderate climates. These animals will simply overheat, tire, and perhaps expire.

Running meant survival as humans expanded their bipedal footprint in what is now known as Eastern Africa. Gatherers on the move found new food and water sources. Hunters chased down game. Christopher McDougall's excellent book, *Born to Run,* introduced the concept of persistence hunting and natural running to a global audience. A majority of his readers were also runners, who discovered a new understanding of what it means to run. Or rather, they became exposed for the very first time to the idea of running injury-free like our stone-age ancestors.

And this is where the brain comes into play. It alone regulates virtually all of our movements, and other bodily activity, when it comes to improving running economy. The brain is exceptionally complex, and so at the risk of oversimplification, it has two key systems that influence the body to make us run so well.

The motor system is how we voluntarily move. (Involuntary actions such as a knee-jerk reflex rely on the spinal cord.) Even before we take that first step on our training run, information from muscles, tendons, joints—especially the feet—is initially sent to the brain for analysis, and immediate decisions are made regarding the most optimal way to run. Specific motor areas on either side of the brain, which control opposite sides of the body, then send messages to muscle fibers that have fine-tuned contraction and relaxation attributes. In making these decisions, the brain considers how much fat and sugar energy is available, the levels of hormones, water, electrolytes, vitamins and other substances necessary to maintain running economy.

The autonomic nervous system keeps many body functions working automatically, such as hormone regulation, breathing, and heart rate. It is housed in the hypothalamus, a small area in the middle of the brain, and consists of a sympathetic and parasympathetic component.

The sympathetic part is our fight or flight mechanism. With help from the spinal cord, it gets us ready to run. Sympathetic activity is most evident leading up to say, race day, with feelings of increased tension preparing the body for what's to come. It makes our muscles stronger, coordinates the release of hormones, constricts the heart for increased blood flow, and deepens breathing to draw more air into the lungs for additional oxygen and expel unwanted carbon dioxide.

The parasympathetic component does virtually the opposite. It calms the body, relaxes the heart, and slows its rate, and prepares the intestines to digest food and absorb nutrients. Basically, we use our parasympathetics for eating and resting.

The hypothalamus is in direct communication with the nearby pituitary gland that oversees the body's hormones, especially those

of the adrenals, which produces an important stress hormone, cortisol. If all goes well, the hypothalamic-pituitary-adrenal axis will be
working hard, and effectively, on race day.

BRAIN-BODY SYNCHRONIZATION (BBS)

As a musician and songwriter, I marvel at the brain's rhythm center,
known as the cerebellum. Positioned near the bottom of the brain,
the cerebellum is one of its more primitive structures. Long before
language, it enabled early humans to develop singing, which played
an important role in survival by strengthening ties among the members of small hunting-and-gathering groups. And it helped develop
the rhythm of running.

Early in my coaching career, I observed that the best runners
effortlessly waltzed along, while average or slower ones struggled to
coordinate their bodies' moving parts. Despite my constant encour-
agement with these slower runners to experience this built-in harmony, such as coordinating their breathing and stride rates, it was
often difficult for them because they had lost their natural rhythm.

I like to think of the running body as a symphony orchestra
with millions of musicians. The brain is the conductor, helping create wonderful sounds and harmonies by the orchestra members. But
if these members are not in synchronization with one another, the
running body will only produce less-than-satisfying music.

When the musicians work together, the synchronization of
body parts—breathing, heart rate, and stride—are in unison and
the result is more efficient running economy. When the music fails,
it's typically due to injury, pain, muscle imbalance, poor nutrition,

and overtraining. There is less organized movement, poor gait, and slower race pace.

The lead runners in a marathon typically are the definition of total body harmony and rhythm. Many of us also feel it during a great workout. It's an example of the synchronization of the entire body. *Entrainment* is the term that's often used to explain the process whereby two or more interacting bodily systems work together in physiological harmony.

With a majority of elite runners, synchronization occurs naturally. These athletes intuitively coordinate heartbeats, inhalation and exhalation, and moving muscles. The body's team effort reflects the brain's innate biofeedback.

Unfortunately, too many runners are out of synch and not in harmony. Impairment of entrainment can occur for many reasons such as mental stress, including pain or anxiety, physical illness, and muscle imbalance. Poor foot function, including wearing the wrong shoes, create disharmony too, as can overtraining even in its early stage.

Seemingly innocuous habits like too much talking to a training partner during a workout, or listening to music that's not in synch with heart, lungs, and stride can negatively impact body rhythms.

Synchronicity was first studied in the 1920s by observing a variety of animals, from cheetahs and leopards, to deer and humans. The common relationships studied were those between breathing rates and foot strikes. By the 1950s, most research was done in Germany (and entrainment may have been one of the so-called secret techniques successfully used by East German and Russian athletes in that era).

Here are three key steps to help improve the brain-body synchronization (BBS), coordinating both breathing and foot strike while running. Those marathoners already going 2:10 or faster probably have optimized their BBS, although some might still be lacking. Even a minor improvement can produce significantly better running economy, potentially taking minutes off one's finishing time. For the rest of the running population—99.9 percent of us—BBS can make dramatic changes in running economy as indicated in a better gait, less injury, and faster training and racing paces.

Step One: The Beat

The first step is to ensure that the brain's basic biofeedback mechanism in the cerebellum is working well. For this, a runner should purchase an inexpensive handheld metronome. This small device provides an audible beat that a runner can adjust to his or her pace. Running to a specific beat might seem easy, but for many, drifting offbeat often happens. Once you start running, adjust the metronome to the beat each time your foot hits the ground.

Employing a metronome for a period of time helps the cerebellum better coordinate movement—for example, by synchronizing one beat for each foot strike. Try it for a week or two by adjusting the rate to match your pace to make sure you can easily hit the ground precisely with each beat. If you have difficulty synchronizing the metronome's beat to your foot hitting the ground, this step will take longer.

Step Two: The Two-Step

Now, instead of relying on the metronome, use your footstrike to maintain the rhythm. This step involves counting both breathing and foot strike. A simple example is breathing in for three strides, then exhale during four strides. This 3:4 relationship would change throughout a run. A 4:5 pattern might exist during warm up and cool down, 2:3 during a race, with a 2:2 in the final "kick."

In most situations, I recommend one more step during exhalation. This ensures ridding the lungs of enough carbon dioxide, and it prevents always landing on the same foot at the onset of inhalation, which can potentially create an imbalance.

Step Three: Shifting Gears

During training and racing, several factors influence pace, gait and effort, especially when running hills. As such, your breathing and stride rate often change. One should be capable of making the appropriate adjustments during the run. It's like shifting gears in a sports car—when properly done, economy improves and speed increases.

During a given run, one should be able to shift from a breath-to-stride pattern of 3:4, to 2:3, then back to 3:4. Practicing will make it easy and almost subconscious, just like shifting gears.

Runners who are in synch can go faster at a lower heart rate. This is due to a more efficient gait and lower oxygen needs.

BRAIN ON PAIN

Pain is a symptom of something abnormal happening. It's an end result with a specific cause. Find and fix it, and the pain typically vanishes. Sometimes the reason for pain is obvious—wearing new racing shoes and getting a bad blister. But often pain seems to just appear one day, as a throbbing hip, knee, low back, or other ache. It may be due to an accumulation of training that is not compensated by adequate rest, or one too many long workouts affecting the low-back muscles. While the pain may be mild or severe, it does not necessarily indicate the extent of the problem—extreme pain can come from a minor muscle imbalance, or a dull ache may be due to a stress fracture.

We sense pain as an emotion deep inside the brain's limbic system, but it may originate in the body as a chemical imbalance, such as a hidden area of inflammation or excess muscle fatigue. Or it could be triggered by nerve endings in a physically damaged tendon, ligament, or joint. It could even be non-specific, such as the ambiguous generalized pain that builds during the course of running a marathon, taxing or overwhelming the whole body at once.

As an emotion, pain is relatively subjective. No two runners feel a seemingly identical knee problem or first metatarsal stress fracture. But pain is not a true sense, like smell, taste, or hearing. Otherwise, it would be much more difficult, or impossible, to control with physical (applying cold), chemical (taking aspirin or other drugs), or mental measures (through hypnosis).

If you are experiencing knee pain, for example, it's not unusual to find yourself automatically rubbing the skin around the joint. This light stimulation of touching or massaging the skin in a painful area sends signals to the brain that can actually block pain processing. Most people do it automatically. Unfortunately, the process works in reverse. Pain disturbs the brain's ability to regulate movement. The result is a disruption of gait with diminished running economy.

Pain reduces the brain's ability to process information coming from the body—it's too busy responding to the high priority of pain. A knee joint screaming in pain literally drowns out this processing of information, disturbing the brain's ability to regulate muscles and movement.

Getting your body out of pain should be a top priority. Otherwise, it can disturb normal movement now, and lead to greater problems down the road. And even if the pain seems minor, it's usually compensated by an altered gait, which not only slows you down and adds more stress to the body, but only delays the inevitable. Through pain, your body is telling you something important—listen.

Pain Meds

Aspirin, ibuprofen (such as Advil), naproxen (such as Aleve), and other nonsteroidal anti-inflammatory drugs (NSAIDs) are commonly used for pain relief. If taking NSAIDs lessens pain, it probably indicates the presence of inflammation, which may be due to an imbalance of dietary fats.

Runners often rely on various types of painkillers, especially NSAIDs, before or after training and racing. One reason is to temporarily mask pain, which can sometimes be successful because inflammation is typically the cause. Many runners think NSAIDS will improve performance; they don't! Just easing the pain during a race may provide some short-term relief, but the negative consequences can be significant. While most of these drugs are not banned in competitive sports, they can cause much more harm than many of the drugs that are banned, in part because they disrupt the normal balance of fats, reduce recovery, and have other unhealthy side effects.

Here is a short list of some potential damaging effects of NSAIDs:

1. They slow the process of recovery and repair in muscles.
2. They cause gut problems, including bleeding in almost everyone taking them (even if it's not noticeable).
3. They can cause muscle dysfunction.
4. They don't necessarily reduce muscle pain associated with training and racing.
5. They can reduce the body's ability to repair joint and bone stress.
6. They can cause kidney damage, especially if one is dehydrated.

7. They can disturb sleep.
8. They may not necessarily reduce all inflammation.
9. They cause immune-system stress.
10. They can actually contribute to injuries.

In addition to NSAIDs for pain control, a second type of drug used for pain relief includes *acetaminophen*. These drugs, mostly non-prescription ones such as Tylenol, don't act by reducing inflammation, and therefore are less likely to interfere with healing and recovery. It's not entirely clear how these drugs work, but liver stress is among the serious side effects. The body needs to break down these drugs in the liver, which requires large amounts of the amino acid cysteine (best obtained in the diet from whey consumption).

Narcotics, such as opiates, are another type of pain reliever. These act in the brain to reduce the sensation of pain and don't affect inflammation. However, they are easily addictive, and their use as a pain reliever wears off as the brain cells become desensitized. Common narcotics prescribed for severe pain include drugs such as codeine, oxycodone (OxyContin) and hydrocodone (Vicodin), relative drugs to morphine and heroin.

Yet another pain-relieving drug is tetrahydrocannabinol, THC, the active component in marijuana. It controls pain by stimulating certain receptors in the brain, similar to those that opiates act upon. THC can stimulate the brain's natural opiates, like endorphins. Many US states and other countries now have medical marijuana laws.

The brain is still a great mystery to neuroscientists and exercise researchers. Medical breakthroughs will continue to shed light on how this organ works. Runners don't need to know all the scientific terms of the brain's regions, or how neurons communicate with one another. At the same time, it is essential not to think of the brain merely as a psychological component of the human body. So when one experiences "hitting the wall," it's not something only occurring inside the mind. Or that the brain can be tricked into doing something against its will, such as doing several extra hill repeats.

In so many ways, the brain is actually the most important part of the runner's body. While many athletes might point to their legs, they should instead direct their attention to the brain. It controls virtually everything. A better functioning brain should be a primary focus of all endurance athletes.

CHAPTER 14

GOING 1:59

The only way to define your limits is by going beyond them.

—ARTHUR CLARKE, author and futurist

The day will soon arrive, probably in the next several years (maybe earlier!) when twenty of the world's fastest marathoners will gather at the starting line inside a large stadium or along a closed-off downtown area of a major city. Billed as "The Race for 1:59," the special made-for-TV event will also shatter the Internet's live-streaming world record of 2.9 million viewers (the royal wedding in England between Prince William and Kate Middleton). A hefty prize purse will be on the line for these handpicked pro runners—a cash payout of $1,000,000 to the winner. The media will call the race "Million-dollar Marathon."

Racing conditions for runners will have to be ideal. Long before these invited runners show up to race, they would have spent months training their bodies specifically for this world-record attempt.

Where will the race take place? Today's marathon locations that draw the strongest fields are determined in large part by television deals, appearance fees and prize money. But these big-city venues, with the possible exception of fast-and-flat Berlin, are not particularly conducive to going 1:59 in the marathon. The event producer will have to consider conditions such as temperature, humidity, and altitude when selecting the perfect racing venue.

Air temperature may be the most significant weather factor that affects racing. The optimal racing temperature is between 40 and 50 degrees Fahrenheit. Outdoor temperature at the start of the race in the low 40s might be best if the finishing temperatures are not above 50 degrees.

In addition to sea level (or lower) locations, and moderate temperatures, the most favorable climate for 1:59 would be one that's relatively dry, but not too dry, as excess dehydration could affect performance.

Ideally, this one-of-a-kind marathon should take place on city streets along a one-mile circuit, or even on an auto racetrack. Staging the event in a stadium on a conventional 400-meter oval track—runners would be racing close to the equivalent of four-and-one-quarter consecutive 10,000-meter races—might be easier to pull off in terms of logistics. But then all those tight turns in the same direction while maintaining a sub-4:35 pace makes a stadium site somewhat impractical.

A staged event on a one-mile loop has many positive attributes, especially regarding the race business. Compared to the city streets, for example, race officials and media would have everything contained in a relatively small area without the issues of traffic control, safety, and securing the course.

This marathon will see many crowd-pleasing things that have been absent from the 26.2-mile race. Because the race is taking place on a closed loop, there might be some jostling and even some pushing among runners. As expected, several rabbits will set a blistering pace. They will drop out by the midway mark, or slightly afterwards. But this could conceivably produce a handful of world-record times for the half-marathon. Still, it's up to each runner to adhere to his own game plan and do his best to ignore the early frontrunners if the pace gets too fast.

To keep the field small and highly competitive, only runners who have gone sub 2:05 in the marathon will be invited to compete. Some of the top pros might have to readjust their racing schedules and sit out some of the big marathons in order to have super fresh legs. Our runners will primarily come from Kenya, Ethiopia, Eritria, and Morocco, with Japan, South Africa, the US, China, Brazil, Russia, and possibly other nations represented. But this all depends on whether these marathoners had made the 2:05 grade.

A handful of runners will be racing barefoot. They will have spent months training without wearing shoes. Every extra ounce, even with superlight racing flats, can make a difference when each second counts. If the marathon course isn't asphalt but a smooth rubberized surface, it will make barefoot running easier on the body. Some of these barefoot runners will have to sacrifice their lucrative shoe endorsement deals, but the opportunity to win one million dollars is a strong monetary incentive to race shoeless. These running rebels would be happy to walk away from their shoe company contracts—not only to capture the grand prize, but also receive millions more in product endorsements over the subsequent years.

Still, there is no guarantee that a 1:59 finish will happen that day. But even if no one accomplishes the feat, the media interest and high television ratings will almost certainly mean that a second race will be held the following year.

There is always the chance that a 1:59 marathon might be set beforehand at an existing race locale, with Berlin the most likely host city since it's a flat course that has already led to a succession of world records. Maybe it will be Boston's "unofficial" course.

Boston Marathon race director Dave McGillivray believes that some great runner is ready and primed for 1:59. "It's got to be the perfect course, with the perfect competition," he says, "with the perfect weather and with the mindset of athletes saying, 'We're going after this.' I don't think we need fifteen years. I think it just has to be the right circumstance. Maybe it needs to be set up. Maybe it's not going to happen on its own."

Appendix A

Why 26.2?

The slow drip of misinformation over multiple generations, colorful myths that unspool from a possible real-life incident, and the obfuscating fog of time affect our understanding of the past. The marathon, as we know it today, is the product of this type of remembrance. As runners, we hold dear the marathon's very own creation myth: a Greek foot-messenger soldier by the name of Pheidippides, was sent from the town of Marathon to Athens to announce that the Persians had been defeated in the Battle of Marathon. He supposedly ran the entire distance without stopping and burst into the Athen senate, uttering these final words: "Masters—victory is ours!" He then collapsed and died due to exhaustion.

The first historical mention of Pheidippides appears in Plutarch's *On the Glory of Athens*, approximately 500 years after the "incident." Give Plutarch his due as an esteemed scholar living in ancient Rome; he didn't have Google or the Internet, and he was merely going by Heraclides Ponticus's lost work.

There's additional confusion as to whether Pheidippedes even existed. Or if that was his real name. Some historians believe that the runner's actual name was Thersipus of Erchius or Eucles.

As for the distance from Marathon to Athens, there's also some ambiguity. Our Greek runner either took the shorter, more mountainous route toward the north with a distance of about 21.4 miles, or the flatter, longer one to the south with a distance of 25.4 miles.

It took a nineteenth century English poet to give now-immortal legs, so to speak, to the myth of Pheidippedes. In 1876, Robert Browning wrote the poem "Pheidippides," which is densely clotted with names, places, and classical allusions that would easily stump any Jeopardy! champion. The lengthy poem's final stanza offers this homage to the Hellenic hero: *Pheidippides happy forever—the noble strong man/ Who could race like a god, bear the face of a god, whom a god loved so well/ He saw the land saved he had helped to save, and was suffered to tell . . .*

When the modern Olympics were birthed two decades later in Athens in 1896, the organizers wanted a unique event that could recall the ancient glory of Greece. That's how the marathon came into existence. The winner of that inaugural Olympic footrace was Spridon Louis, a Greek water-carrier, who won in a time of 2:24:52. The total distance, however, was 24.85 miles.

So how did the marathon end up becoming 26.2 miles? Why were those extra 1.3 miles added? At the 1908 Olympic Games in London, the marathon distance was lengthened to twenty-six miles to cover the ground from Windsor Castle to White City stadium, with another 385 yards tacked on so the race could finish in front of King Edward VII's royal box.

Twenty-six miles and 385 yards wasn't immediately adopted as the official marathon race distance. It often fluctuated between twenty-four and twenty-five miles. The first Chicago marathons in the early 1900s were twenty-five miles. Nor was there any consensus as to what a marathon actually was. Popular races billed as marathons or "modified marathons," some with distances as short as ten or twelve miles, took place in cities such as New York, Philadelphia, and Los Angeles.

For the next Olympics in 1912, the marathon was shortened to 40.2 kilometers (24.98 miles) and revised again to 42.75 kilometers (26.56 miles) for the 1920 Olympics. In fact, of the first seven Olympic marathons, there were six different marathon distances between 40 kilometers and 42.75 kilometers.

It wasn't until the 1924 Olympics in Paris that the International Amateur Athletic Federation (IAAF) established the official marathon distance as 26.2 miles. According to IAAF Rule 240, "The distance converted into miles, 26.2187, has been rounded to 26.22 in the table (a difference of about 2 yards)."

Had the marathon retained its original distance from the first modern Olympic Games, the first sub-two hour marathon would have happened by now, and most likely, it would have occurred some time in the late 1990s.

Appendix B

1:59 Marathon Candidates

O
ne cannot write a book about the 1:59 marathon without suggesting likely candidates. Runners from Kenya and Ethiopia, as most will obviously expect to see, top my list.

To arrive at my list, I looked at the top fifty marathon times over the last three years, considered the best all-time performances, factored in personal, course, and world records, and paid particular attention to those who made this exclusive list more than twice. I also looked at the recurrence of exceptional races—the "what have you done lately?" factor, which can be negatively influenced by injuries, poor health, and overtraining. Just as important is consistency, an important feature because a fast marathon is experience-based—those who have run a few hard races and survived well have learned a lot about how to make significant improvements.

Of course, any elite marathoner can have a breakthrough race and run 1:59. This includes all of the runners listed here, along with relatively unknowns who occasionally turn in strong performances. For many other runners, the issue is whether they have already peaked, are prematurely past their prime, or are too injured to return to their past greatness. Sometimes a victory is accomplished by someone who successfully returns from a period of poor performance. Or, not infrequently, a mildly overtrained marathoner who hits a race just right, and whose PR is measured in minutes not seconds.

Here are my top three candidates:

-Geoffrey Mutai (Kenya). At thirty-two years old, he is riding a long period of great racing (2009-present). His 2011 Boston Marathon was 2:03:02, and he also has a 58:55 half (2013).
-Wilson Kipsang (Kenya). The thrity-one-year-old owns an impressive string of wins between 2009 and 2013, including a world record of 2:03:23. Four of his marathon times are in top fifty (2 in the top 5), and he also has a 58:59 half.
-Dennis Kimetto (Kenya). At thirty years old, he had great performances primarily between 2011-2013, including a 2:03:45 in Chicago (2013). Two of his best marathon times are in the top fifty (top 11), and he has a 59:14 half marathon.

Now, the runner-ups:

-Emmanuel Mutai (Kenya). A couple of breakthrough races in 2011 and 2013. Two of his marathon times are in the top fifty.
-Haile Gebrselassie (Ethiopia). His amazing career as a top candidate may have ended in 2010.
-Eliud Kipchoge (Kenya). At age thirty, and with great middle distance speed and a 59:25 half marathon, his 2013 showing n Berlin of 2:04:05 might mean his better times are ahead.
-Ayele Absehero (Ethiopia). A debut in Dubai of 2:04:23 in 2012. Perhaps good things ahead if he can remain healthy.
-James Kipsang Kwambai (Kenya). Appeared to peak in 2009 with a 2:04:27 marathon and 59:09 half-marathon
-Tesgaye Asefa (Ethiopia). At only nineteen years young, his debut in Dubai in 2014 at 2:04:32 makes him a potential candidate, but his

next few races will tell more. He may actually be too young, that is, unless he stays healthy.

-Tsegay Kebede (Ethiopia). With all the credentials, he may have peaked in 2012 (Chicago 2:04:38).

-Lelisa Desisa Benti (Ethiopia). Another great debut in Dubai— 2:04.45 in 2013. A great middle-distance career, only twenty-four years young, another wait-and-see candidate.

-Yemane Adhane Tsegay (Ethiopia). His 2:04:48 in 2012 may have been a peak.

-Berhanu Shiferaw (Ethiopia). His 2:04:48 in 2013 (Dubai) may have been a peak.

-Tadese Tola (Ethiopia). May have peaked early in 2013 with his 2:04:49 in Dubai.

Virtually dozens of other great runners are potential 1:59 candidates. Almost all are East Africans. At one time, Ryan Hall (2:04:58 in Boston 2011 and the fastest marathon ever run by an American) seemed like the guy to go 1:59. But after several injuries and a disappointing Boston 2014 (2:17:50), that may no longer be the case unless he can return to form.

Obviously, there are many other elite, world-class marathoners who probably deserve inclusion on this list. Feel free to suggest a potential 1:59 candidate, or several, by contacting me through my website (PhilMaffetone.com).